INTERMITTENT
FASTING FOR
WOMEN OVER 50

A comprehensive guide to eat healthy,lose weight,get fit with 28-day meal plan

KERI K. HUEY

TABLE OF CONTENTS

INTRODUCTION

Jennifer, who lives in the heart of the charming community of Meadow Grove, found herself at a crossroads as she approached her fifties. She sensed a need for change, a desire to revive her health and well-being while surrounded by the eternal beauty of nature. She had no idea that a simple cookbook would become the start for a life-changing trip.

One ordinary day, while wandering through the shelves of the town's quaint bookstore, Jennifer stumbled upon a book that would soon reshape her life. The title beckoned her: "Intermittent Fasting for Women Over 50." Drawn by the promise of a rejuvenated life, she eagerly acquired the cookbook, setting in motion a series of events that would not only impact her but also resonate with the women in her community.

Unveiling the Secrets Within

As she delved into the pages of the cookbook, she discovered a wealth of knowledge curated by experts in women's health. The book tailored intermittent fasting to the unique needs of women in their 50s, addressing hormonal changes, metabolism, and overall well-being. Each recipe seemed crafted to fuse nutrition and flavor, offering a roadmap for a healthier lifestyle.

Dawn of a New Routine

With the cookbook in hand, Jennifer embarked on her intermittent fasting journey. The carefully designed meal plans and fasting protocols became her compass, guiding her through a new daily routine. The concept of embracing periods of fasting wasn't just about restriction; it was a mindful approach to eating, allowing her body to experience periods of rest and rejuvenation.

Culinary Adventures and Rediscovered Tastes

The cookbook unfolded a kaleidoscope of culinary adventures for Jennifer. From nourishing breakfasts to savory dinners and delightful snacks, each recipe became a celebration of health and flavor. Gone were the days of mundane meals; instead, Jennifer savored the rediscovery of tastes that fueled not only her body but also her zest for life.

Radiance from Within

As Jennifer persisted on her intermittent fasting odyssey, the effects rippled through her life. She felt a surge of energy that defied the stereotypes associated with aging. Her skin glowed with newfound radiance, a testament to the rejuvenating power of nourishing her body with wholesome, well-timed meals. Jennifer became living proof that age was no barrier to vitality.

The Quiet Revolution

In a town where routines rarely changed, Jennifer's transformation didn't go unnoticed. Friends and acquaintances marveled at her newfound vitality, prompting them to inquire about the secret behind her radiant glow. With genuine enthusiasm, Jennifer began sharing her story, attributing her rejuvenation to the cookbook that had become her trusted guide.

Empowering the Women of Meadow Grove

Word of Jennifer's journey spread like wildfire, igniting a quiet revolution in Meadow Grove. The women in the community, inspired by her radiant health, embraced the intermittent fasting lifestyle. The local bookstore struggled to keep the cookbook in stock as women of all ages sought the keys to unlocking their own vitality.

From Cookbook to Community

Her impact extended beyond her immediate circle. Recognizing the power of communal support, she initiated gatherings where women could share their experiences, exchange recipe variations, and encourage one another. What began as a personal journey had evolved into a vibrant community of empowered women, all nourishing their bodies and spirits with the wisdom found in the cookbook.

Paying It Forward

Jennifer's commitment to empowering women didn't stop at her immediate community. With a sense of purpose, she reached out to neighboring towns, organizing workshops and seminars to share the transformative potential of intermittent fasting. Her mission was clear: to pay forward the gift of revitalized health and well-being.

A Legacy of Wellness

As she entered the later years of her 50s, she reflected on the journey that had begun with a simple cookbook. The legacy she left behind wasn't just one of personal transformation but a testament to the collective power of women supporting each other on the path to wellness. Meadow Grove had become a haven of radiance, where age was embraced as a journey, not a limitation.

Beyond the Cookbook

Her story, woven into the fabric of Meadow Grove, exemplifies the transformative power of embracing change in the pursuit of well-being. The cookbook that sparked her journey became a beacon of inspiration for women seeking a vibrant, fulfilling life. Through sharing her experience and building a community, Jennifer not only revitalized her own health but also became a catalyst for a wellness revolution that touched the lives of women far beyond the borders of her quaint town.

CHAPTER 1:

Understanding Intermittent Fasting

Intermittent Fasting (IF) is a dietary approach characterized by alternating cycles of eating and fasting, with periods of food consumption followed by deliberate periods of abstaining. The concept revolves around timing rather than specific food restrictions, making it a flexible and sustainable option for many individuals.

Understanding Intermittent Fasting involves recognizing its various methods, the most common being the 16/8 method where one fasts for 16 hours and eats within an 8-hour window. Other approaches include the 5:2 method, involving normal eating for five days and reduced caloric intake for two non-consecutive days, and the Eat-Stop-Eat method, which involves a 24-hour fast once or twice a week.

Scientifically, intermittent fasting triggers several physiological responses. During the fasting phase, the body depletes stored glucose, prompting the utilization of fat stores for energy. This process is associated with benefits such as improved insulin sensitivity, reduced inflammation, and potential weight loss. Moreover, fasting periods may stimulate the production of ketones, molecules with neuroprotective properties.

Understanding the relevance of Intermittent Fasting to specific demographics, such as women over 50, requires consideration of age-related changes in metabolism and hormonal fluctuations. Tailoring fasting plans to accommodate these factors is essential for optimizing health outcomes.

The History of Intermittent Fasting

The history of Intermittent Fasting (IF) dates back centuries and has roots in various cultural and religious practices. Fasting has been observed in different forms across civilizations as a means of spiritual purification, self-discipline, and even a way to promote physical health.

One of the earliest instances of fasting can be traced to ancient Greece, where the renowned physician Hippocrates prescribed abstinence from food as a method to allow the body to heal itself. In ancient Rome, the philosopher Seneca advocated for periodic fasting as a means of developing self-control and resilience.

Intermittent Fasting also has deep ties to religious traditions. Practices such as Ramadan in Islam involve daily fasting from sunrise to sunset, emphasizing spiritual reflection and self-discipline. Similarly, Lent in Christianity incorporates fasting as a way to commemorate the forty days Jesus spent fasting in the desert.

In more recent times, scientific interest in Intermittent Fasting has grown. Research in the mid-20th century discovered the potential health benefits of calorie restriction and intermittent fasting. The 21st century has seen a surge in popularity, with various fasting methods gaining recognition for their purported effects on metabolic health, weight management, and longevity.

The historical journey of Intermittent Fasting reflects a convergence of cultural, religious, and scientific influences, shaping it into the diverse and dynamic dietary practice it is today.

The Benefits of Intermittent Fasting for Women Over 50

Intermittent Fasting (IF) holds several potential benefits for women over 50, offering a holistic approach to health and well-being.

1. Hormonal Balance: As women age, hormonal fluctuations, particularly during menopause, can lead to challenges such as weight gain and mood swings. IF has been shown to positively influence hormone levels, potentially mitigating these issues and promoting hormonal balance.

2. Weight Management: Weight gain is a common concern for women in their 50s. IF can be an effective strategy for weight management by promoting fat utilization for energy during fasting periods and supporting a healthy metabolism.

3. Cardiovascular Health: IF has been associated with improvements in cardiovascular health markers such as blood pressure, cholesterol levels, and reduced inflammation. These benefits are particularly crucial for women over 50 who may be at a higher risk of heart-related issues.

4. Cognitive Function: IF has shown promise in supporting cognitive function and reducing the risk of neurodegenerative diseases. For women over 50, maintaining cognitive health is vital, and IF may contribute to enhanced brain function.

5. Insulin Sensitivity: Aging is often linked to decreased insulin sensitivity, leading to an increased risk of Type 2 diabetes. IF may improve insulin sensitivity, helping to regulate blood sugar levels and reduce the risk of diabetes.

Different Types of Intermittent Fasting

Intermittent Fasting (IF) encompasses various approaches, each characterized by distinct fasting and eating periods. Understanding the different types allows individuals to choose a method that aligns with their lifestyle, preferences, and health goals.

1. 16/8 Method (Time-Restricted Eating): One of the most popular forms of IF, the 16/8 method involves a daily fasting window of 16 hours and an eating window of 8 hours. For example, an individual might eat between 12:00 pm and 8:00 pm, fasting from 8:00 pm to 12:00 pm the next day.

2. 5:2 Diet (Modified Fasting): This approach involves consuming a regular diet for five days a week and significantly reducing caloric intake (around 500-600 calories) on two non-consecutive days. This intermittent calorie restriction aims to achieve health benefits without daily fasting.

3. Eat-Stop-Eat: This method incorporates 24-hour fasting periods once or twice a week. For instance, someone might eat dinner at 7:00 pm one day and then abstain from eating until 7:00 pm the following day.

4. Alternate-Day Fasting: This more rigorous approach involves alternating between days of regular eating and days of significant caloric restriction or complete fasting. Some variations permit a small amount of calories (around 500) on fasting days.

5. Warrior Diet: Inspired by the eating patterns of ancient warriors, this method involves consuming small amounts of raw fruits and vegetables during the day and having one large meal at night within a 4-hour eating window.

6. OMAD (One Meal A Day): As the name suggests, OMAD involves eating only one substantial meal a day, typically within a one-hour window. The rest of the day is spent fasting.

7. Spontaneous Meal Skipping: A more flexible approach, individuals can opt to skip meals spontaneously, adapting IF to their schedule. This might involve occasionally skipping breakfast or dinner.

Understanding the nuances of these different types of Intermittent Fasting enables individuals to choose an approach that suits their lifestyle and health objectives.

It's essential to approach IF with balance, ensuring that nutritional needs are met during eating windows.

Getting Started with Intermittent Fasting

Embarking on the journey of Intermittent Fasting (IF) requires thoughtful preparation and a gradual transition to this dietary approach. Here's a guide on getting started:

1. Mental Preparation: Before diving into IF, it's crucial to mentally prepare for a shift in eating habits. Understand the goals behind intermittent fasting, whether it's weight management, improved metabolism, or other health benefits. This mental readiness contributes significantly to adherence.

2. Setting Realistic Goals: Define clear and realistic goals for your intermittent fasting journey. Whether it's starting with a specific fasting window, achieving weight loss, or improving overall well-being, having measurable objectives provides motivation and direction.

3. Choosing the Right Method: Explore the various types of IF and choose one that aligns with your lifestyle. The 16/8 method is a popular starting point, offering an 8-hour eating window and 16-hour fasting period. Experiment with different methods to find the one that suits your routine and preferences.

4. Creating a Fasting Schedule: Establish a fasting schedule that integrates seamlessly into your daily life. Consider factors such as work, family commitments, and social engagements when deciding on your fasting and eating windows. Consistency is key to adapting to IF successfully.

5. Gradual Transition: For beginners, a gradual transition into intermittent fasting is often more sustainable. Start by delaying your first meal or skipping a snack, gradually extending the fasting window over days or weeks until you reach your desired schedule.

6. Hydration is Key: Stay well-hydrated during fasting periods. Water, herbal teas, and black coffee are generally permitted during fasting and can help manage hunger and support overall well-being.

7. Monitoring Hunger and Energy Levels: Pay attention to your body's signals. It's normal to experience hunger initially, but listen to your body's cues and adjust your fasting window accordingly. If energy levels drop significantly, consider revisiting your fasting approach.

8. Seeking Professional Guidance: Consult with healthcare professionals or a registered dietitian before starting IF, especially if you have underlying health conditions. They can provide personalized advice based on your individual needs.

Getting started with intermittent fasting is a personal journey that requires patience and self-awareness. By approaching it with a well-thought-out plan and a gradual adjustment, individuals can increase their likelihood of successfully incorporating IF into their lifestyle.

Finding Your Ideal Fasting Window

1. Lifestyle and Schedule: Evaluate your daily commitments, work hours, and social engagements. Choose a fasting window that aligns with your routine to ensure consistency. If you have a 9-to-5 job, for instance, a 16/8 method with an eating window from noon to 8:00 pm might suit your schedule.

2. Personal Preferences: Consider your natural eating habits and preferences. Some individuals prefer having a substantial breakfast, while others find it easier to skip breakfast and have a larger meal later in the day. Tailor your fasting window to what feels most natural and sustainable for you.

3. Energy Levels and Productivity: Pay attention to your energy levels and productivity at different times of the day. If you find that you are more alert and focused in the morning, you may want to schedule your eating window accordingly. Conversely, if you are more active and hungry in the evening, adjust your fasting window to accommodate this.

4. Social Considerations: Be mindful of social occasions and family meals. If you enjoy dinner gatherings or breakfast meetings, plan your eating window to coincide with these events. Flexibility is key to integrating IF into your social life without feeling restricted.

5. Experimentation and Adaptation: Intermittent Fasting is not a one-size-fits-all approach. Experiment with different fasting windows to understand what suits you best. Start with a 12-hour fasting window and gradually extend it based on your comfort level. Be open to adjusting as needed.

6. Listen to Your Body: Pay attention to hunger cues and how your body responds to different fasting windows. If you consistently feel fatigued or overly hungry during a specific fasting period, consider modifying it. The goal is to find a balance that supports both your health goals and well-being.

7. Consistency is Key: Once you identify your ideal fasting window, strive for consistency. Regularity in your eating and fasting patterns helps your body adjust and enhances the effectiveness of Intermittent Fasting.

Remember that finding the ideal fasting window is a dynamic process. It may evolve as your lifestyle changes or as you become more accustomed to intermittent fasting. Listen to your body, be flexible, and enjoy the benefits of a fasting window that aligns with your unique needs.

Tips for Staying Focused During Fasting

1. Stay Hydrated: Adequate hydration is crucial during fasting. Water helps stave off dehydration and can also help manage feelings of hunger. Herbal teas and black coffee are also permissible and can add variety to your fluid intake.

2. Mindful Distractions: Engage in activities that keep your mind occupied and distracted from thoughts of food. Whether it's work, hobbies, reading, or spending time with loved ones, finding fulfilling distractions can make fasting periods more manageable.

3. Gradual Adjustment: If you're new to Intermittent Fasting, consider a gradual adjustment to longer fasting periods. Starting with shorter windows and slowly extending them over time allows your body and mind to adapt.

4. Balanced Nutrition: Ensure that your meals within the eating window are nutrient-dense and well-balanced. A combination of protein, healthy fats, and complex carbohydrates can help maintain energy levels and keep you feeling satisfied.

5. Listen to Your Body: Pay attention to hunger cues and energy levels. If you feel overly fatigued or hungry, consider adjusting your fasting window or incorporating small, nutritious snacks during the fasting period.

6. Quality Sleep: Prioritize quality sleep, as fatigue and lack of rest can make fasting more challenging. Establish a consistent sleep routine to support overall well-being and mental focus during fasting.

7. Social Support: Share your Intermittent Fasting journey with friends or family who can provide encouragement. Having a support system can make the process more enjoyable and foster a sense of accountability.

8. Mindful Eating: When breaking your fast, practice mindful eating. Chew slowly, savor your food, and be present during meals. This can enhance satisfaction and prevent overeating, contributing to a positive fasting experience.

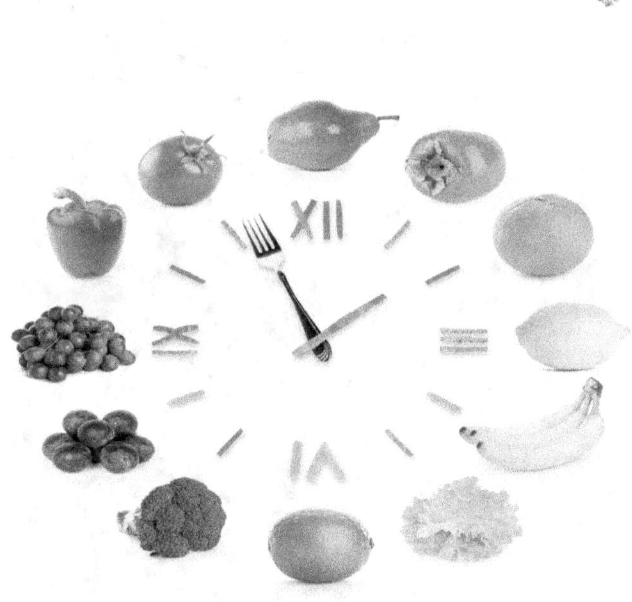

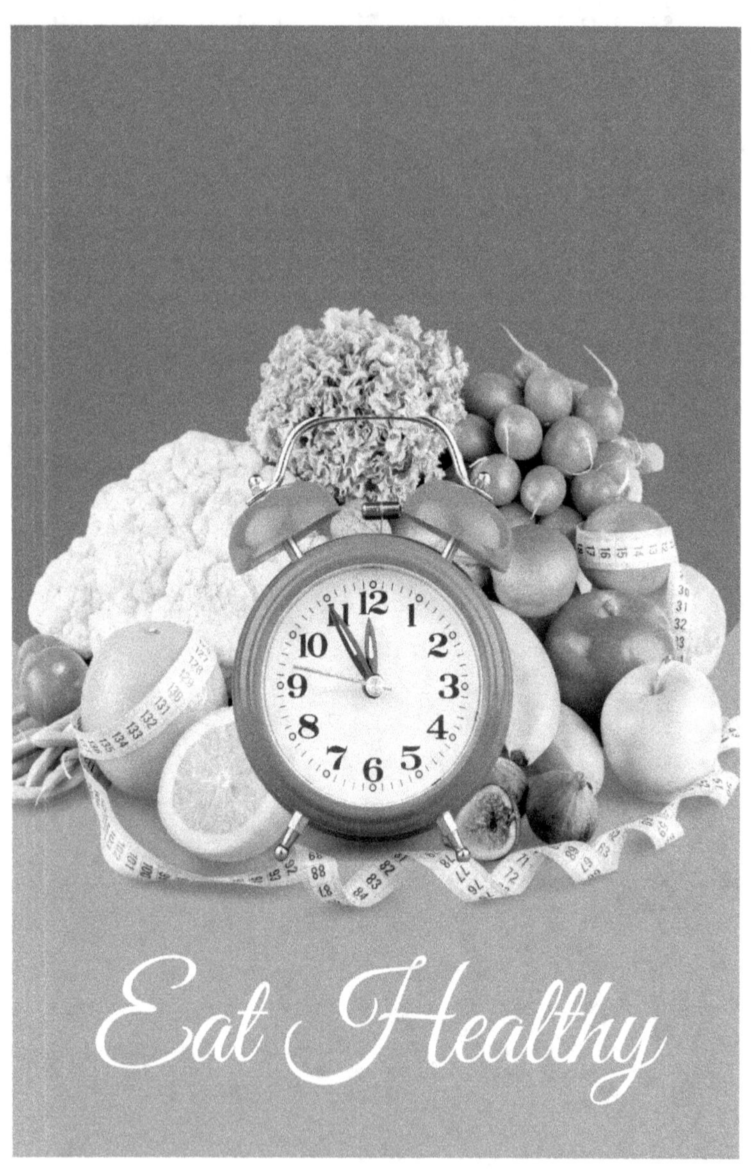
Eat Healthy

CHAPTER 2:

HEALTH AND LIFESTYLE FACTORS

Intermittent Fasting and Aging

Intermittent Fasting (IF) holds promise in addressing age-related challenges. As individuals age, metabolic changes and hormonal fluctuations can impact health and weight management. IF may counteract these effects, promoting metabolic flexibility, improved insulin sensitivity, and potential cognitive benefits. Research suggests that IF might contribute to healthy aging by optimizing cellular processes and reducing inflammation, providing a holistic approach to wellness in the later stages of life. However, it's essential to approach IF with consideration of individual health conditions and consult healthcare professionals for personalized guidance.

The Hormonal Benefits of Intermittent Fasting

Intermittent Fasting (IF) exerts notable hormonal benefits, particularly in regulating insulin and human growth hormone (HGH). During fasting periods, insulin sensitivity improves, helping to stabilize blood sugar levels and reduce the risk of Type 2 diabetes. Simultaneously, IF triggers an increase in HGH, crucial for metabolism, muscle maintenance, and overall vitality. This hormonal surge contributes to enhanced fat metabolism and may facilitate muscle preservation. IF's positive impact on hormones extends to promoting cellular repair and reducing inflammation, showcasing its potential as a holistic approach to health and well-being. It's essential to note that individual responses may vary, and consulting healthcare professionals is advisable before adopting IF, especially for those with existing health conditions.

Intermittent Fasting and Chronic Conditions

Research suggests that IF may positively impact conditions such as Type 2 diabetes, cardiovascular issues, and inflammation. By improving insulin sensitivity, IF can help regulate blood sugar levels, reducing diabetes risk. Additionally, IF's impact on cardiovascular health markers, like cholesterol and blood pressure, may contribute to managing heart-related conditions. While promising, it's crucial for individuals with chronic conditions to consult healthcare professionals before incorporating IF into their routine, ensuring a safe and tailored approach to support overall well-being.

Weight Loss and Intermittent Fasting

The practice of intermittent fasting (IF) has gained appeal as a viable weight reduction approach. IF promotes the body to use stored fat for energy by enforcing regulated fasting intervals, hence boosting fat reduction. The limited eating windows also limit calorie intake, which contributes to overall energy balance. IF may boost metabolism, increase insulin sensitivity, and aid in long-term weight control. Furthermore, the method's adaptability supports a variety of lifestyles, making it a viable option for people looking for successful and flexible weight reduction solutions. However, it's critical to approach IF with a balanced mindset, including healthy meals during eating windows and talking with healthcare specialists to assess its suitability for specific health objectives.

Intermittent Fasting and Mental Health

The technique of intermittent fasting has been shown to have potential advantages for mental health in addition to its physical effects. Fasting induces biological processes that may have an impact on brain health, such as the creation of brain-derived neurotrophic factor (BDNF), which is linked to cognitive function and mood control. IF may also aid in cellular repair processes, lowering oxidative stress and inflammation, which may have an influence on mental health. While practicing IF, some people experience greater attention, mental clarity, and emotional stabilization. However, it is critical to approach IF with an awareness of individual requirements, since significant changes in eating habits may have varying effects on mood and energy levels. To guarantee a safe and customized approach to intermittent fasting, it is recommended that you consult with a healthcare expert, particularly if you have pre-existing mental health concerns.

The Connection Between Intermittent Fasting and Brain Function

Intermittent Fasting for Reducing Anxiety and Depression

Intermittent Fasting (IF) may play a role in reducing anxiety and depression symptoms by influencing various biological processes. Fasting periods can trigger the release of brain-derived neurotrophic factor (BDNF), linked to improved mood and cognitive function. IF also modulates inflammation and oxidative stress, factors associated with mental health conditions. Additionally, the metabolic benefits of IF, such as improved insulin sensitivity, may positively impact neurotransmitter regulation. While some individuals report mental health improvements with IF, it's crucial to approach it cautiously, considering individual responses and consulting healthcare professionals. Lifestyle modifications, including dietary changes like IF, can be one aspect of a comprehensive approach to mental well-being, which may also include therapy, medication, and other interventions based on individual needs.

Intermittent Fasting for Cognitive Function Enhancement

Intermittent Fasting (IF) shows promise in enhancing cognitive function through various physiological mechanisms. Fasting periods stimulate the production of brain-derived neurotrophic factor (BDNF), a protein associated with cognitive health, learning, and memory. IF also promotes autophagy, a cellular cleaning process that eliminates damaged cells and proteins, potentially supporting brain health. The metabolic switch during fasting, where the body utilizes ketones for energy, may offer neuroprotective benefits. Improved insulin sensitivity, a result of IF, is linked to better brain function. Some studies suggest that IF may reduce oxidative stress and inflammation in the brain, contributing to cognitive resilience. While research is ongoing, anecdotal evidence and preliminary studies propose that IF could be a valuable lifestyle approach for those seeking to optimize cognitive performance. However, individual responses vary, and it's important to adopt IF cautiously, considering overall health and consulting healthcare professionals, especially for those with underlying conditions or concerns about the potential impact on cognitive health.

Combining Intermittent Fasting with Other Diets

Mediterranean Diet and Intermittent Fasting

The combination of the Mediterranean Diet and Intermittent Fasting (IF) represents a holistic approach to nutrition that promotes both health and sustainable weight management.

Mediterranean Diet:

The Mediterranean Diet is renowned for its emphasis on whole, nutrient-dense foods that reflect the traditional dietary patterns of countries bordering the Mediterranean Sea. This diet is rich in fruits, vegetables, whole grains, legumes, and healthy fats like olive oil. It includes moderate amounts of fish, poultry, and dairy, with limited red meat consumption. The Mediterranean Diet is associated with numerous health benefits, including reduced risk of heart disease, improved cognitive function, and better weight management.

Intermittent Fasting:

IF involves alternating between periods of eating and fasting, with various methods like the 16/8 method or the 5:2 approach. It focuses on when to eat rather than specific food restrictions, allowing for flexibility in food choices during eating windows.

Synergies of Mediterranean Diet and IF:
1. Nutrient-Dense Eating: The Mediterranean Diet's focus on whole, plant-based foods complements the nutritional principles of IF. During eating windows, individuals following this combination can enjoy a variety of nutrient-dense foods.

2. Improved Metabolic Health: Both the Mediterranean Diet and IF have been linked to improved metabolic health. The Mediterranean Diet's emphasis on healthy fats and IF's impact on insulin sensitivity work synergistically to support overall metabolic function.

3. Sustainable Weight Management: The combination of these two approaches promotes a sustainable and balanced way of eating. IF can enhance the metabolic benefits of the Mediterranean Diet, potentially aiding in weight loss or weight maintenance.

4. Long-Term Health Benefits: Both the Mediterranean Diet and IF have demonstrated long-term health benefits, including reduced inflammation, improved cardiovascular health, and enhanced cognitive function.

Adopting the Mediterranean Diet in conjunction with Intermittent Fasting offers a flexible and well-rounded lifestyle approach to nutrition.

Renal diet and intermittent fasting

The integration of a Renal Diet with Intermittent Fasting (IF) requires careful attention and individualized planning, particularly for those with renal problems. A Renal Diet is intended to maintain and promote renal function by controlling food intake, notably salt, potassium, and phosphorus.

Renal Diet:
A Renal Diet typically involves controlling the amount of protein, sodium, and other minerals to alleviate the workload on the kidneys. It often includes limited intake of high-potassium and high-phosphorus foods while ensuring an adequate supply of essential nutrients.

Intermittent Fasting:
IF involves alternating between eating and fasting periods. While some research suggests potential benefits for metabolic health, weight management, and inflammation reduction, individuals with kidney issues must approach IF cautiously due to its potential impact on hydration and electrolyte balance.

Considerations for Combining Renal Diet and IF:
1. Fluid Balance: Proper hydration is crucial for kidney health. IF may lead to decreased water intake during fasting periods, which can potentially affect fluid balance. Individuals on a Renal Diet need to ensure adequate hydration.

2. Nutrient Intake: Individuals following a Renal Diet should be mindful of their nutrient intake during eating windows in IF. It's essential to maintain a balance of nutrients while adhering to Renal Diet restrictions.

3. Consulting Healthcare Professionals: Given the specialized nature of Renal Diets and potential implications of fasting on kidney function, it is crucial for individuals with kidney concerns to consult healthcare professionals before incorporating IF into their routine.

4. Personalized Approach: The combination of a Renal Diet and IF requires a highly individualized approach. Factors such as the severity of kidney issues, overall health, and medications must be considered to develop a safe and effective plan.

Keto Diet and Intermittent Fasting

The combination of the Ketogenic Diet (Keto) and Intermittent Fasting (IF) has gained popularity for its potential synergies in promoting weight loss and metabolic health.

The Keto Diet:

The Keto Diet is characterized by high fat, moderate protein, and very low carbohydrate intake, leading the body into a state of ketosis. In ketosis, the body shifts from using glucose as its primary energy source to burning fat, which may result in weight loss and improved energy levels. The Keto Diet emphasizes foods like meat, fish, eggs, dairy, nuts, and healthy oils while restricting carbohydrates.

Intermittent Fasting:

IF involves cycling between periods of eating and fasting. The fasting periods can range from a few hours to several days, with the aim of utilizing stored fat for energy during the fasting window. Common IF methods include the 16/8 method, where one fasts for 16 hours and eats within an 8-hour window, or the 5:2 method, involving regular eating for five days and reduced caloric intake on two non-consecutive days.

Synergies of Keto and IF:

1. Enhanced Fat Burning: Combining Keto and IF amplifies the utilization of stored fat for energy. When the body is in ketosis during fasting periods, it efficiently burns fat for fuel.

2. Stabilized Blood Sugar: The low-carb nature of the Keto Diet helps regulate blood sugar levels, and IF further supports insulin sensitivity, collectively contributing to metabolic health.

3. Improved Focus and Mental Clarity: Both Keto and IF have been associated with cognitive benefits. Ketones produced during ketosis are considered a cleaner source of energy for the brain, potentially enhancing mental focus.

4. Weight Loss: The dual approach of restricting carbohydrate intake and incorporating fasting windows can accelerate weight loss by promoting fat metabolism.

Intermittent Fasting for Long-Term Health

Practicing intermittent fasting (IF) has evolved as a lifestyle option with long-term health advantages that go beyond immediate benefits. One important characteristic is its ability to boost metabolic wellness. IF has been linked to increased insulin sensitivity, which may lower the incidence of Type 2 diabetes and help with long-term blood sugar control.

Additionally, IF has shown positive effects on cardiovascular health markers. Studies suggest that it may contribute to lowering blood pressure, improving cholesterol levels, and reducing inflammation, factors crucial for long-term heart health.

IF's impact on cellular repair and autophagy, the body's process of cleaning out damaged cells, is another aspect with potential long-term benefits. These processes are linked to aging and may contribute to increased longevity and improved overall health.

Furthermore, IF may aid in weight management over the long term. By promoting fat utilization for energy during fasting periods and helping control caloric intake, IF offers a sustainable approach to maintaining a healthy weight.

Cognitive benefits are also noteworthy. IF has been associated with increased levels of brain-derived neurotrophic factor (BDNF), a protein linked to cognitive function, mood regulation, and potentially reduced risk of neurodegenerative diseases.

However, it's crucial to approach IF with a balanced perspective. Nutrient-rich, well-rounded meals during eating windows are essential to ensure that the body receives adequate nourishment. Moreover, consulting with healthcare professionals is advisable, especially for individuals with pre-existing health conditions, to tailor an IF approach that aligns with their unique needs.

Paleo Diet and Intermittent Fasting

The Paleo diet combined with Intermittent Fasting (IF) creates a synergistic approach to health and fitness by combining ancestral feeding habits with intentional fasting periods. The Paleo diet emphasizes complete, unprocessed foods, similar to our hypothesized hunter-gatherer ancestors' diet. It focuses on lean meats, fruits and vegetables, nuts, and seeds while avoiding grains, legumes, and processed foods.

Pairing the Paleo diet with Intermittent Fasting capitalizes on the evolutionary concept of feast and famine. During the eating windows, individuals following the Paleo diet consume nutrient-dense, natural foods. The fasting periods complement this approach by promoting metabolic flexibility, encouraging the utilization of stored fat for energy, and potentially enhancing the benefits of both dietary strategies.

The Paleo diet's focus on quality nutrients supports sustained energy levels, and when combined with intermittent fasting, it may aid in weight management and metabolic health. Moreover, the duo's potential to reduce inflammation and improve insulin sensitivity aligns with both the Paleo philosophy and the goals of intermittent fasting.

However, it's essential to approach this combination with individual considerations. Balancing nutrient intake during eating windows is crucial to meet dietary needs, especially given the exclusion of certain food groups in the Paleo diet. Consulting with healthcare professionals is advisable, especially for individuals with specific health conditions, to ensure a well-rounded and personalized approach.

Intermittent Fasting and Heart Health

Intermittent Fasting (IF) has garnered attention for its potential positive impact on heart health, offering a multifaceted approach to cardiovascular well-being. Several aspects of IF contribute to its potential benefits for the heart.

One significant factor is its influence on weight management. IF often leads to a reduction in overall caloric intake, aiding in weight loss and the maintenance of a healthy weight. Excess weight is a known risk factor for cardiovascular diseases, and by promoting weight loss, IF may help mitigate this risk.

IF has also demonstrated the ability to improve metabolic health by enhancing insulin sensitivity. Improved insulin function is associated with better control of blood sugar levels, which is crucial for reducing the risk of Type 2 diabetes—a condition linked to heart disease.

Moreover, IF has been linked to favorable changes in cardiovascular risk factors. Studies suggest that it may contribute to lowering blood pressure, reducing levels of harmful LDL cholesterol, and improving triglyceride levels. These factors collectively play a pivotal role in cardiovascular health and the prevention of heart-related issues.

Additionally, IF's impact on inflammation may contribute to its cardiovascular benefits. Chronic inflammation is a key player in the development of heart disease, and IF has shown potential in reducing inflammatory markers, fostering a more heart-protective environment.

However, it's essential to approach IF with a balanced perspective, ensuring that individuals maintain a nutrient-rich diet during eating windows to support overall health. Consulting with healthcare professionals, especially for those with existing heart conditions, is advisable to tailor an IF approach that aligns with individual health needs.

Galveston diet and Intermittent fasting

The Galveston Diet and Intermittent Fasting (IF) represent two distinct yet compatible approaches to health and weight management, combining principles of nutrition and strategic fasting.

The Galveston Diet, designed by Dr. Mary Claire Haver, is specifically tailored for women in perimenopause and menopause. It emphasizes anti-inflammatory foods, healthy fats, and lean proteins while limiting refined carbohydrates and sugars. This dietary approach aims to support hormonal balance, mitigate inflammation, and promote overall well-being during a stage of life often associated with metabolic changes.

When integrated with Intermittent Fasting, the Galveston Diet can become a powerful tool for women's health. IF's structured fasting periods complement the Galveston Diet by tapping into the body's natural ability to burn fat for energy. This aligns with the diet's focus on nutrient-dense foods and supports the metabolic shifts associated with perimenopause and menopause.

The combination of the Galveston Diet and IF can contribute to weight management, improved insulin sensitivity, and potential benefits for cardiovascular health. By incorporating fasting windows, individuals may enhance the diet's impact on inflammation and promote cellular repair, aspects integral to both approaches.

As with any dietary strategy, individual responses may vary, and it's crucial to approach these methods with consideration for personal health needs. Consulting healthcare professionals, especially for those with specific health conditions or concerns, ensures a tailored and safe approach.

Intermittent fasting and Golo diet

Intermittent Fasting (IF) and the GOLO Diet represent distinct but potentially complementary approaches to weight management and overall health.

IF involves cycling between periods of eating and fasting, with various methods like the 16/8, 5:2, or Eat-Stop-Eat. It focuses on the timing of meals to optimize metabolism, improve insulin sensitivity, and promote fat utilization for energy during fasting periods.

The GOLO Diet, on the other hand, is a comprehensive dietary plan that emphasizes whole foods, portion control, and managing insulin levels. It places a particular emphasis on choosing foods that do not spike blood sugar, promoting sustained energy and weight loss.

When integrated, these approaches can create a synergistic effect. IF's strategic fasting periods align with GOLO's emphasis on insulin management, potentially enhancing the diet's impact on blood sugar levels. The controlled eating windows during IF can complement GOLO's focus on portion control and nutrient-dense foods.

Both approaches share a common goal of supporting metabolic health and weight loss. IF offers flexibility in timing, while the GOLO Diet provides a structured nutritional framework. Combining these strategies may contribute to improved insulin sensitivity, enhanced fat metabolism, and sustainable weight management.

Gut Health and Intermittent Fasting

The relationship between gut health and Intermittent Fasting (IF) is a subject of growing interest in the field of nutrition. The gut, often referred to as the "second brain," plays a crucial role in overall health, influencing digestion, immune function, and even mental well-being.

IF may positively impact gut health through various mechanisms. One key aspect is its potential to promote a balanced gut microbiome. The fasting periods in IF allow the gut to undergo periods of rest, facilitating the growth of beneficial bacteria and promoting microbial diversity. This, in turn, may contribute to improved digestion, nutrient absorption, and a strengthened immune system.

Moreover, IF's influence on inflammation may extend to the gut. Chronic inflammation is associated with various gastrointestinal issues, and by reducing overall inflammation, IF could potentially alleviate some gut-related concerns.

The regulation of gut hormones is another significant factor. IF has been shown to influence hormones like ghrelin and leptin, which play roles in hunger regulation and satiety. This hormonal balance may contribute to a more regulated appetite and better digestion.

However, it's crucial to approach IF with consideration for individual responses. Some individuals may experience temporary digestive discomfort during fasting periods, and it's essential to listen to one's body and make adjustments accordingly.

Maintaining a balanced, nutrient-dense diet during eating windows is vital for gut health. Incorporating fiber-rich foods, prebiotics, and probiotics supports a healthy gut microbiome. Hydration is equally important, as water helps maintain gut function and overall digestive health.

Intermittent Fasting and Immune System

Intermittent Fasting (IF) has emerged as a lifestyle approach with potential benefits for the immune system, the body's defense against infections and diseases. Research suggests that IF may contribute to immune system modulation through various mechanisms.

One key factor is the impact of IF on inflammation. Chronic inflammation is linked to immune system dysfunction and various health issues. IF has been shown to reduce markers of inflammation, creating an environment that may support overall immune function.

Autophagy, a cellular process triggered during fasting, is another aspect relevant to immune health. Autophagy involves the removal of damaged cells and cellular components, contributing to cellular renewal. This process may play a role in optimizing immune cell function.

IF's influence on the gut microbiome is also noteworthy. The gut is a significant component of the immune system, and a balanced gut microbiome is crucial for immune health. IF's potential to promote microbial diversity and a healthy gut environment may indirectly support immune function.

Moreover, IF's impact on metabolic health aligns with immune system support. Improved insulin sensitivity and weight management, often associated with IF, may contribute to overall metabolic health, reducing the risk of immune-related disorders.

It's important to note that individual responses to IF may vary, and there is a need for more research to fully understand the complex relationship between IF and the immune system. Additionally, a balanced approach is essential, ensuring that individuals maintain proper nutrition and hydration during eating windows to support immune health.

Skin Health and Intermittent Fasting

The technique of intermittent fasting has sparked interest not just for its potential effect on internal health, but also for its impact on exterior aspects such as skin health. While research in this area is still in its early stages, there are various ways in which IF may help to preserve good skin.

One notable factor is the potential reduction in oxidative stress. During fasting periods, the body may experience a decrease in oxidative stress, which is linked to aging and skin damage. By promoting cellular repair mechanisms, IF may contribute to a more youthful and vibrant complexion.

IF's influence on inflammation is also significant for skin health. Chronic inflammation is associated with various skin conditions, and IF has been shown to reduce inflammatory markers. This may contribute to a calmer, clearer complexion and potentially alleviate symptoms of inflammatory skin conditions.

Additionally, IF's impact on insulin sensitivity and blood sugar levels may play a role in skin health. Elevated blood sugar levels are associated with skin aging and acne. IF's ability to regulate insulin levels may contribute to better control of blood sugar, potentially benefiting skin appearance.

Hydration is crucial for skin health, and during fasting periods, individuals are encouraged to stay well-hydrated. Proper hydration supports skin elasticity, reducing the likelihood of dryness and promoting a healthy complexion.

While IF may offer potential benefits for skin health, it's essential to approach it with a balanced perspective. Maintaining a nutrient-dense diet during eating windows is vital to provide the skin with the necessary vitamins and minerals for optimal health.

Individual responses to IF may vary, and factors such as skin type and existing skin conditions should be considered. Consulting with dermatologists or skincare professionals is advisable for personalized advice, especially for those with specific skin concerns or conditions.

Intermittent Fasting and Energy Levels

The practice of IF has been shown to have a considerable impact on energy levels, offering a novel way to control and enhance everyday vitality. Several interrelated systems govern the connection between IF and energy..

One of the primary ways IF impacts energy levels is through the body's utilization of fuel sources. During fasting periods, the body shifts from relying on glucose derived from food to tapping into stored fat for energy. This metabolic switch, known as ketosis, can contribute to more stable and sustained energy levels throughout the day.

IF has been associated with improvements in mitochondrial function. Mitochondria are the energy-producing powerhouses within cells. Enhanced mitochondrial function may lead to increased energy production, supporting overall vitality.

IF's potential to regulate blood sugar levels is another factor influencing energy. By promoting improved insulin sensitivity, IF helps prevent rapid spikes and crashes in blood sugar, contributing to more consistent energy levels. This is particularly beneficial for individuals prone to energy fluctuations after meals.

Cognitive function is closely tied to energy levels, and IF has shown promise in supporting brain health. The production of brain-derived neurotrophic factor (BDNF) during fasting periods may contribute to enhanced mental clarity, focus, and overall cognitive function, positively impacting energy levels.

While many individuals report increased energy levels and improved alertness during fasting periods, it's essential to approach IF with consideration for individual responses. Some people may experience an adjustment period as the body adapts to a new eating schedule.

Maintaining proper hydration during fasting periods is crucial for sustaining energy levels. Water, herbal teas, and black coffee are typically allowed during fasting and can contribute to overall hydration.

Intermittent Fasting and Exercise

Fasting on occasion (IF) and exercise have a fascinating interaction since both improve general health and well-being. Combining IF with a structured workout program may maximize the advantages of both approaches.

One of the notable advantages of exercising during fasting periods is the potential to optimize fat utilization for energy. When the body is in a fasted state, it relies on stored fat for fuel, making it an opportune time for activities that promote fat burning, such as cardio and high-intensity interval training (HIIT). This can be particularly beneficial for individuals aiming for weight management and improved metabolic health.

Strength training, including weightlifting, can also complement IF. Some individuals prefer to schedule their weightlifting sessions during eating windows to ensure they have sufficient nutrients for muscle recovery. The protein-rich meals consumed after workouts contribute to muscle repair and growth.

IF's impact on insulin sensitivity aligns with the benefits of exercise. Combining both practices may amplify the improvement in insulin function, potentially reducing the risk of Type 2 diabetes and promoting better blood sugar control.

The timing of exercise in relation to fasting windows is a personal choice. Some individuals prefer to exercise during fasting periods, capitalizing on the potential fat-burning benefits, while others find it more comfortable to work out during eating windows.

It's crucial to pay attention to individual energy levels and preferences. While some people thrive on fasting and exercising, others may find it more suitable to break their fast before engaging in physical activity. Staying hydrated is essential during both fasting and exercise to support overall performance and well-being.

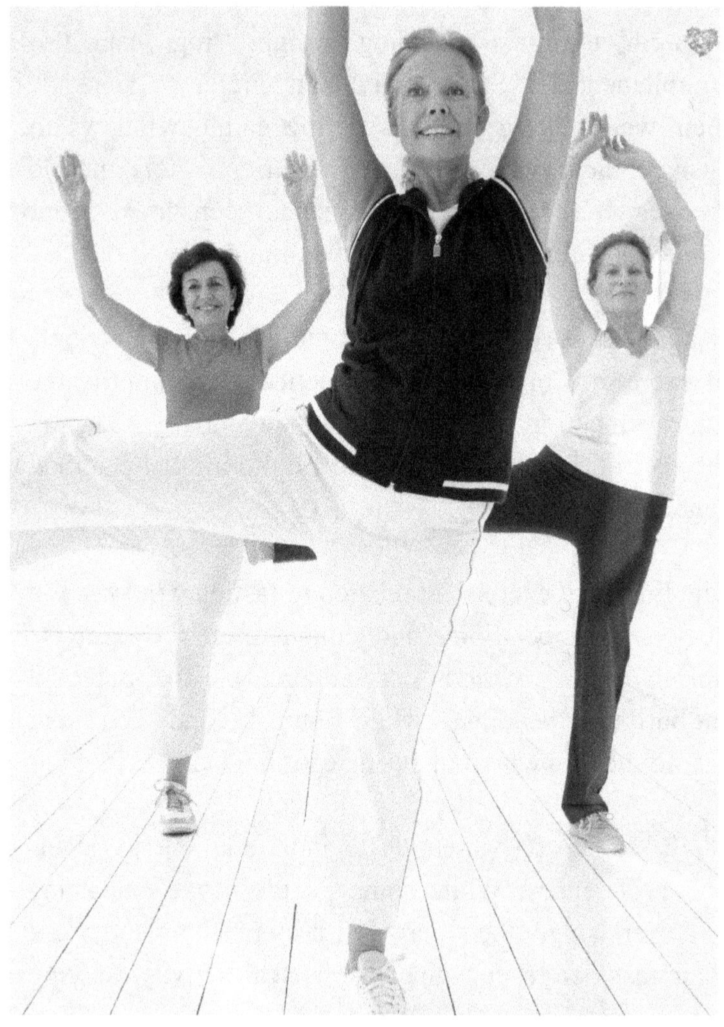

CHAPTER 3:

BREAKFAST RECIPES

Avocado and Smoked Salmon Toast:

Ingredients:
- 1 slice whole-grain bread
- 1/2 avocado, mashed
- 2 oz smoked salmon
- 1 tsp lemon juice
- Salt and pepper to taste

Instructions:
1. Toast the whole-grain bread.
2. Spread mashed avocado on the toast.
3. Top with smoked salmon.
4. Drizzle with lemon juice and season with salt and pepper.

Nutrition approx.

Calories	Protein	Carbohydrates	Fat
250	15g	20g	12g

- Prep Time: 5 minutes
- Cook Time: 2 minutes
- Serves: 1

Greek Yogurt Parfait:

Ingredients:
- 1 cup Greek yogurt
- 1/2 cup mixed berries (strawberries, blueberries, raspberries)
- 1 tbsp chia seeds
- 1 tbsp honey

Instructions:
1. In a glass, layer Greek yogurt with mixed berries.
2. Sprinkle chia seeds on top.
3. Drizzle with honey.

Nutrition approx.

Calories	Protein	Carbohydrates	Fat
300	20g	30g	12g

- Prep Time: 5 minutes
- Serves: 1

Vegetable Omelet:

Ingredients:
- 2 eggs
- 1/4 cup diced bell peppers
- 1/4 cup diced tomatoes
- 1/4 cup chopped spinach
- 1 tbsp olive oil
- Salt and pepper to taste

Instructions:

1. In a bowl, whisk eggs and season with salt and pepper.

2. Heat olive oil in a pan over medium heat.

3. Add bell peppers, tomatoes, and spinach to the pan.

4. Pour whisked eggs over the vegetables and cook until set.

Nutrition approx.

Calories	Protein	Carbohydrates	Fat
250	15g	5g	18g

- Prep Time: 10 minutes
- Cook Time: 5 minutes
- Serves: 1

Quinoa Breakfast Bowl:

Ingredients:
- 1/2 cup cooked quinoa
- 1/4 cup almond milk
- 1/2 banana, sliced
- 1 tbsp almond butter
- 1 tbsp shredded coconut

Instructions:

1. In a bowl, combine cooked quinoa and almond milk.

2. Top with sliced banana, almond butter, and shredded coconut.

Nutrition approx.

Calories	Protein	Carbohydrates	Fat
300	8g	40g	12g

- Prep Time: 5 minutes
- Serves: 1

Spinach and Feta Egg Muffins:

Ingredients:
- 3 eggs
- 1/2 cup chopped spinach
- 1/4 cup crumbled feta cheese

- 1/4 cup diced tomatoes
- Salt and pepper to taste

Instructions:

1. Preheat the oven to 350°F (175°C).

2. In a bowl, whisk eggs and add chopped spinach, feta cheese, and tomatoes.

3. Pour the mixture into muffin cups.

4. Bake for 15-20 minutes until eggs are set.

Nutrition approx.

Calories	Protein	Carbohydrates	Fat
200	15g	5g	14g

- Prep Time: 10 minutes
- Cook Time: 15-20 minutes
- Serves: 2-3 (depending on muffin cup size)

Overnight Chia Seed Pudding:

Ingredients:

- 2 tbsp chia seeds
- 1/2 cup almond milk
- 1/2 tsp vanilla extract
- 1/2 cup mixed berries
- 1 tbsp sliced almonds

Instructions:

1. In a jar, combine chia seeds, almond milk, and vanilla extract.

2. Stir well, cover, and refrigerate overnight.

3. In the morning, top with mixed berries and sliced almonds.

Nutrition approx.

Calories	Protein	Carbohydrates	Fat
220	6g	20g	12g

- Prep Time: 5 minutes (plus overnight refrigeration)
- Serves: 1

Apple Cinnamon Oatmeal:

Ingredients:
- 1/2 cup rolled oats
- 1/2 cup almond milk
- 1/2 apple, diced
- 1/2 tsp cinnamon
- 1 tbsp chopped walnuts

Instructions:
1. In a saucepan, combine rolled oats and almond milk.

2. Cook over medium heat until oats are tender.

3. Stir in diced apple, cinnamon, and top with chopped walnuts.

Nutrition approx.

Calories	Protein	Carbohydrates	Fat
280	7g	35g	14g

- Prep Time: 10 minutes
- Cook Time: 5 minutes
- Serves: 1

Almond Flour Pancakes:

Ingredients:
- 1/2 cup almond flour
- 2 eggs
- 1/4 cup almond milk
- 1/2 tsp baking powder
- 1/2 tsp vanilla extract

Instructions:

1. In a bowl, whisk together almond flour, eggs, almond milk, baking powder, and vanilla extract.

2. Heat a non-stick skillet and pour batter to make pancakes.

3. Cook until bubbles form, then flip and cook the other side.

Nutrition approx.

Calories	Protein	Carbohydrates	Fat
320	12g	8g	25g

- Prep Time: 10 minutes
- Cook Time: 10 minutes
- Serves: 2

Cottage Cheese and Pineapple Bowl:

Ingredients:
- 1/2 cup low-fat cottage cheese
- 1/2 cup fresh pineapple chunks
- 1 tbsp shredded coconut
- 1 tbsp chopped mint leaves

Instructions:
1. In a bowl, combine cottage cheese and fresh pineapple.

2. Sprinkle shredded coconut and garnish with chopped mint.

Nutrition approx.

Calories	Protein	Carbohydrates	Fat
180	15g	20g	5g

- Prep Time: 5 minutes
- Serves: 1

Sweet Potato and Kale Breakfast Hash:

Ingredients:
- 1 cup sweet potatoes, diced
- 1 cup kale, chopped
- 2 eggs
- 1 tbsp olive oil
- Salt and pepper to taste

Instructions:

1. In a skillet, heat olive oil and add diced sweet potatoes.

2. Cook until sweet potatoes are tender, then add chopped kale.

3. Create wells in the mixture and crack eggs into them.

4. Cover and cook until eggs are done to your liking.

Nutrition approx.

Calories	Protein	Carbohydrates	Fat
300	12g	30g	15g

- Prep Time: 15 minutes
- Cook Time: 15 minutes
- Serves: 2

Berry and Spinach Smoothie:

Ingredients:

- 1 cup spinach
- 1/2 cup mixed berries (strawberries, blueberries, raspberries)
- 1/2 banana
- 1/2 cup Greek yogurt
- 1/2 cup water or almond milk

Instructions:

1. Blend spinach, mixed berries, banana, Greek yogurt, and water/almond milk until smooth.
2. Pour into a glass and enjoy.

Nutrition approx.

Calories	Protein	Carbohydrates	Fat
200	15g	30g	5g

- Prep Time: 5 minutes
- Serves: 1

Egg and Vegetable Breakfast Wrap:

Ingredients:

- 2 eggs, scrambled
- 1 whole-grain wrap

- 1/2 cup sautéed vegetables (bell peppers, onions, mushrooms)
    - 1 tbsp salsa

Instructions:

1. Fill the whole-grain wrap with scrambled eggs, sautéed vegetables, and salsa.

2. Roll it up and enjoy.

Nutrition apprx.

Calories	Protein	Carbohydrates	Fat
300	15g	30g	12g

- Prep Time: 10 minutes
- Cook Time: 5 minutes
- Serves: 1

Quinoa and Fruit Salad:

Ingredients:
- 1/2 cup cooked quinoa
- 1/2 cup mixed fresh fruits (berries, kiwi, mango)
- 1 tbsp chopped nuts (almonds, walnuts)
- 1 tbsp honey

Instructions:

1. Combine cooked quinoa, mixed fruits, chopped nuts, and drizzle with honey.

2. Mix well and serve.

Nutrition apprx.

Calories	Protein	Carbohydrates	Fat
250	6g	40g	8g

- Prep Time: 15 minutes
- Serves: 1

Peanut Butter and Banana Toast:

Ingredients:
- 1 slice whole-grain bread
- 2 tbsp natural peanut butter
- 1/2 banana, sliced
- Drizzle of honey

Instructions:
1. Toast the whole-grain bread.
2. Spread peanut butter on the toast and top with banana slices.
3. Drizzle with honey.

Nutrition apprx.

Calories	Protein	Carbohydrates	Fat
280	10g	30g	15g

- Prep Time: 5 minutes

- Serves: 1

Salmon and Cream Cheese Bagel:

Ingredients:
- 1 whole-grain bagel, toasted
- 2 oz smoked salmon
- 2 tbsp cream cheese
- Capers and fresh dill for garnish

Instructions:

1. Spread cream cheese on the toasted whole-grain bagel.

2. Top with smoked salmon and garnish with capers and fresh dill.

Nutrition approx.

Calories	Protein	Carbohydrates	Fat
300	20g	30g	12g

- Prep Time: 10 minutes
- Serves: 1

Blueberry Almond Oatmeal:

Ingredients:
- 1/2 cup rolled oats
- 1/2 cup almond milk

- 1/2 cup fresh or frozen blueberries
- 1 tbsp almond butter
- 1 tsp honey

Instructions:

1. Cook rolled oats with almond milk until tender.

2. Stir in blueberries, almond butter, and drizzle with honey.

Nutrition approx.

Calories	Protein	Carbohydrates	Fat
280	8g	40g	10g

- Prep Time: 7 minutes
- Cook Time: 5 minutes
- Serves: 1

Veggie and Feta Scramble:

Ingredients:

- 2 eggs, beaten
- 1/2 cup diced bell peppers
- 1/4 cup diced tomatoes
- 2 tbsp crumbled feta cheese
- 1 tbsp chopped fresh basil

Instructions:

1. In a pan, sauté bell peppers and tomatoes until softened.

2. Add beaten eggs and scramble.

3. Stir in feta cheese and fresh basil.

Nutrition approx.

Calories	Protein	Carbohydrates	Fat
250	15g	10g	16g

- Prep Time: 10 minutes
- Cook Time: 5 minutes
- Serves: 1

Apple Walnut Overnight Oats:

Ingredients:

- 1/2 cup rolled oats
- 1/2 cup almond milk
- 1/2 apple, diced
- 1 tbsp chopped walnuts
- 1/2 tsp cinnamon

Instructions:

1. Mix rolled oats with almond milk, diced apple, chopped walnuts, and cinnamon.

2. Refrigerate overnight and enjoy in the morning.

Nutrition approx.

Calories	Protein	Carbohydrates	Fat
260	8g	35g	12g

- Prep Time: 5 minutes (plus overnight refrigeration)
- Serves: 1

Greek Yogurt and Granola Parfait:

Ingredients:

- 1 cup Greek yogurt
- 1/4 cup granola
- 1/2 cup mixed berries
- Drizzle of honey

Instructions:

1. In a glass, layer Greek yogurt with granola and mixed berries.

2. Drizzle with honey and serve.

Nutrition approx.

Calories	Protein	Carbohydrates	Fat
300	20g	30g	12g

- Prep Time: 5 minutes
- Serves: 1

Spinach and Mushroom Frittata:

Ingredients:
- 3 eggs
- 1/2 cup chopped spinach
- 1/4 cup sliced mushrooms
- 1/4 cup grated Parmesan cheese
- Salt and pepper to taste

Instructions:
1. Preheat the oven to 350°F (175°C).

2. Whisk eggs and mix with chopped spinach, sliced mushrooms, and Parmesan cheese.

3. Pour the mixture into a greased baking dish and bake until set.

Nutrition approx.

Calories	Protein	Carbohydrates	Fat
280	18g	5g	20g

- Prep Time: 15 minutes
- Cook Time: 20 minutes
- Serves: 2

Banana Almond Smoothie Bowl:

Ingredients:
- 1 frozen banana

- 1/2 cup almond milk
- 1 tbsp almond butter
- Toppings: sliced bananas, chia seeds, and granola

Instructions:

1. Blend frozen banana, almond milk, and almond butter until smooth.

2. Pour into a bowl and top with sliced bananas, chia seeds, and granola.

Nutrition approx.

Calories	Protein	Carbohydrates	Fat
250	5g	30g	14g

- Prep Time: 5 minutes
- Serves: 1

Mediterranean Egg Muffins:

Ingredients:
- 4 eggs, beaten
- 1/2 cup cherry tomatoes, halved
- 1/4 cup feta cheese, crumbled
- 2 tbsp black olives, sliced
- Fresh oregano for garnish

Instructions:

1. Preheat the oven to 350°F (175°C).

2. In a bowl, mix beaten eggs with cherry tomatoes, feta cheese, and black olives.

3. Pour the mixture into muffin cups and bake until eggs are set.

4. Garnish with fresh oregano.

Nutrition approx.

Calories	Protein	Carbohydrates	Fat
280	18g	6g	20g

- Prep Time: 15 minutes
- Cook Time: 15 minutes
- Serves: 2-3

Mango Coconut Chia Pudding:

Ingredients:
- 2 tbsp chia seeds
- 1/2 cup coconut milk
- 1/2 cup fresh mango, diced
- 1 tbsp shredded coconut

Instructions:
1. In a jar, mix chia seeds and coconut milk.

2. Refrigerate for a few hours or overnight.

3. Top with fresh mango and shredded coconut before serving.

Nutrition approx.

Calories	Protein	Carbohydrates	Fat
220	5g	20g	15g

- Prep Time: 5 minutes (plus chilling time)
- Serves: 1

Turkey and Veggie Breakfast Wrap:

Ingredients:
- 1 whole-grain wrap
- 3 slices turkey breast
- 1/4 cup baby spinach
- 1/4 cup cherry tomatoes, sliced
- 1 tbsp Greek yogurt

Instructions:
1. Lay the turkey slices on the whole-grain wrap.
2. Add baby spinach and cherry tomatoes.
3. Drizzle with Greek yogurt, wrap, and enjoy.

Nutrition approx.

Calories	Protein	Carbohydrates	Fat
260	20g	25g	10g

- Prep Time: 7 minutes
- Serves: 1

Almond and Berry Protein Pancakes:

Ingredients:
- 1/2 cup almond flour
- 2 eggs
- 1/4 cup almond milk
- 1/2 cup mixed berries
- 1 tbsp almond butter

Instructions:

1. Mix almond flour, eggs, and almond milk to make pancake batter.

2. Cook spoonfuls of batter on a skillet until golden.

3. Top with mixed berries and a dollop of almond butter.

Nutrition approx.

Calories	Protein	Carbohydrates	Fat
300	15g	15g	20g

- Prep Time: 10 minutes
- Cook Time: 10 minutes
- Serves: 2

Pumpkin Spice Smoothie:

- Ingredients:
  - 1/2 cup canned pumpkin puree

- 1/2 banana
- 1/2 cup almond milk
- 1/2 tsp pumpkin spice
- 1 tbsp chia seeds

- Instructions:

1. Blend pumpkin puree, banana, almond milk, and pumpkin spice until smooth.

2. Stir in chia seeds and let it sit for a few minutes before enjoying.

Nutrition approx.

Calories	Protein	Carbohydrates	Fat
220	5g	30g	10g

- Prep Time: 5 minutes
- Serves: 1

Caprese Avocado Toast:

- Ingredients:
    - 1 slice whole-grain bread
    - 1/2 avocado, mashed
    - 1/2 cup cherry tomatoes, halved
    - Fresh basil leaves
    - Balsamic glaze for drizzling

- Instructions:

1. Toast the whole-grain bread.

2. Spread mashed avocado on the toast and top with cherry tomatoes and basil.

3. Drizzle with balsamic glaze.

Nutrition approx.

Calories	Protein	Carbohydrates	Fat
250	5g	30g	15g

- Prep Time: 7 minutes
- Serves: 1

Chocolate Protein Smoothie Bowl:

Ingredients:

- 1/2 cup Greek yogurt
- 1/2 banana
- 1 scoop chocolate protein powder
- Toppings: sliced strawberries, shredded coconut, and cacao nibs

Instructions:

1. Blend Greek yogurt, banana, and chocolate protein powder until smooth.

2. Pour into a bowl and top with sliced strawberries, shredded coconut, and cacao nibs.

Nutrition approx.

Calories	Protein	Carbohydrates	Fat
280	25g	20g	10g

- Prep Time: 5 minutes
- Serves: 1

Cinnamon Apple Quinoa Bowl:

- Ingredients:
- 1/2 cup cooked quinoa
  - 1/2 apple, diced
  - 1 tbsp chopped walnuts
  - 1/2 tsp cinnamon
  - 1 tbsp maple syrup

- Instructions:
1. Mix cooked quinoa with diced apple, chopped walnuts, cinnamon, and maple syrup.
2. Warm in the microwave if desired before serving.

Nutrition approx.

Calories	Protein	Carbohydrates	Fat
260	6g	40g	8g

- Prep Time: 7 minutes
- Serves: 1

Smoked Salmon and Cream Cheese Bagel:

Ingredients:
- 1 whole-grain bagel, toasted
- 2 oz smoked salmon
- 2 tbsp cream cheese
- Capers and fresh dill for garnish

Instructions:

1. Spread cream cheese on the toasted whole-grain bagel.

2. Top with smoked salmon and garnish with capers and fresh dill.

Nutrition approx.

Calories	Protein	Carbohydrates	Fat
300	20g	30g	12g

- Prep Time: 10 minutes
- Serves: 1

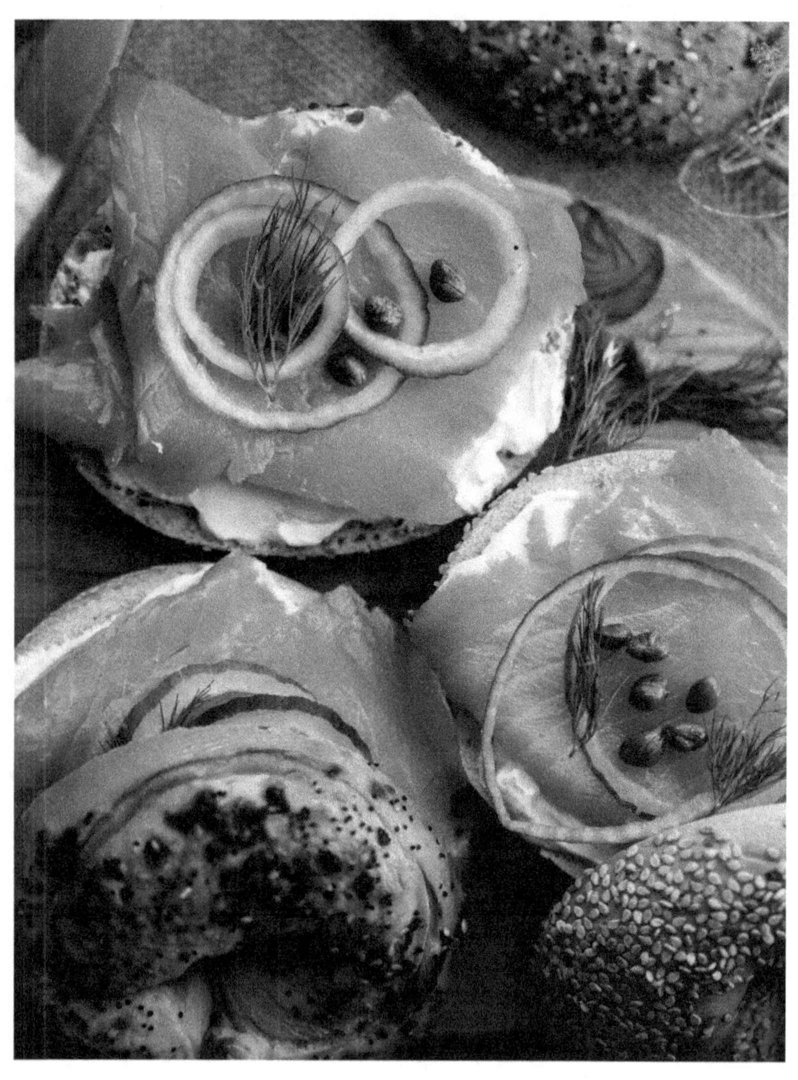

CHAPTER 4:

FISH AND SEAFOOD RECIPES

Grilled Lemon Herb Salmon:

Ingredients:
- 2 salmon filets
- 1 lemon, sliced
- 2 tbsp olive oil
- 1 tsp dried thyme
- Salt and pepper to taste

Instructions:
1. Preheat the grill.
2. Rub salmon filets with olive oil, thyme, salt, and pepper.
3. Place lemon slices on top of each filet.
4. Grill for 8-10 minutes or until salmon is cooked through.

Nutrition approx.

Calories	Protein	Fat
300	30g	15g

- Prep Time: 10 minutes
- Cook Time: 10 minutes
- Serves: 2

Shrimp and Asparagus Stir-Fry:

Ingredients:
- 1 lb shrimp, peeled and deveined
- 1 bunch asparagus, trimmed
- 2 tbsp soy sauce
- 1 tbsp sesame oil
- 1 tsp ginger, minced

Instructions:

1. In a pan, stir-fry shrimp and asparagus in sesame oil.

2. Add soy sauce and ginger, cook until shrimp is pink and asparagus is tender.

Nutrition approx.

Calories	Protein	Fat
250	25g	10g

- Prep Time: 15 minutes
- Cook Time: 10 minutes
- Serves: 4

Baked Cod with Mediterranean Salsa:

Ingredients:
- 4 cod filets
- 1 cup cherry tomatoes, halved
- 1/2 cup Kalamata olives, chopped
- 1/4 cup red onion, finely chopped
- 2 tbsp olive oil
- 1 tbsp balsamic vinegar

Instructions:
1. Preheat the oven.
2. Season cod filets and bake until cooked through.
3. Mix tomatoes, olives, red onion, olive oil, and balsamic vinegar for salsa.
4. Serve cod with Mediterranean salsa on top.

Nutrition approx.

Calories	Protein	Fat
280	30g	15g

- Prep Time: 15 minutes
- Cook Time: 20 minutes
- Serves: 4

Lemon Garlic Butter Shrimp:

Ingredients:
- 1 lb large shrimp, peeled and deveined
- 3 tbsp butter
- 4 cloves garlic, minced
- 1 lemon, juiced
- 2 tbsp fresh parsley, chopped

Instructions:
1. In a pan, melt butter and sauté garlic until fragrant.
2. Add shrimp and cook until pink.
3. Stir in lemon juice and parsley.

Nutrition approx.

Calories	Protein	Fat
220	25g	12g

- Prep Time: 10 minutes
- Cook Time: 8 minutes
- Serves: 3

Tuna and White Bean Salad:

Ingredients:
- 2 cans tuna, drained
- 1 can white beans, rinsed and drained
- 1 cucumber, diced

- 1/4 cup red onion, finely chopped
- 2 tbsp olive oil
- 1 tbsp red wine vinegar
- Salt and pepper to taste

Instructions:

1. In a bowl, combine tuna, white beans, cucumber, and red onion.

2. Drizzle with olive oil and red wine vinegar.

3. Season with salt and pepper, toss well.

Nutrition approx.

Calories	Protein	Fat
320	35g	15g

- Prep Time: 15 minutes
- Serves: 4

Seared Scallops with Lemon Garlic Butter:

Ingredients:

- 1 lb sea scallops
- 2 tbsp olive oil
- 3 cloves garlic, minced
- Zest of 1 lemon
- 2 tbsp fresh parsley, chopped

Instructions:

1. Pat scallops dry and season with salt and pepper.

2. Heat olive oil in a pan and sear scallops until golden brown.

3. Add minced garlic, lemon zest, and parsley. Cook for an additional minute.

Nutrition approx.

Calories	Protein	Fat
250	25g	10g

- Prep Time: 10 minutes
- Cook Time: 5 minutes
- Serves: 3

Cajun Baked Catfish:

Ingredients:
- 4 catfish filets
- 2 tbsp Cajun seasoning
- 1 tbsp olive oil
- 1 lemon, sliced

Instructions:

1. Preheat the oven.

2. Rub catfish filets with Cajun seasoning and olive oil.

3. Place lemon slices on top and bake until fish flakes easily.

Nutrition approx.

Calories	Protein	Fat
280	30g	12g

- Prep Time: 15 minutes
- Cook Time: 20 minutes
- Serves: 4

Coconut Shrimp Curry:

Ingredients:
- 1 lb shrimp, peeled and deveined
- 1 can coconut milk
- 2 tbsp red curry paste
- 1 bell pepper, sliced
- 1 cup snap peas

Instructions:

1. In a pan, combine coconut milk and red curry paste. Simmer.

2. Add shrimp, bell pepper, and snap peas. Cook until the shrimp is pink.

Nutrition approx.

Calories	Protein	Fat

300	25g	20g

- Prep Time: 15 minutes
- Cook Time: 15 minutes
- Serves: 3

Garlic Herb Baked Halibut:

Ingredients:
- 4 halibut filets
- 3 tbsp olive oil
- 3 cloves garlic, minced
- 1 tbsp fresh thyme, chopped
- Salt and pepper to taste

Instructions:
1. Preheat the oven.
2. Place halibut filets on a baking sheet.
3. Mix olive oil, minced garlic, and thyme. Brush over halibut.
4. Bake until the fish is opaque and flakes easily.

Nutrition approx.

Calories	Protein	Fat
300	30g	15g

- Prep Time: 10 minutes

- Cook Time: 15 minutes
- Serves: 4

Lemon Dill Grilled Swordfish:

Ingredients:
- 4 swordfish steaks
- Zest and juice of 1 lemon
- 2 tbsp fresh dill, chopped
- 2 tbsp olive oil

Instructions:
1. Preheat the grill.
2. Mix lemon zest, lemon juice, dill, and olive oil.
3. Brush the mixture over swordfish steaks and grill until cooked.

Nutrition approx.

Calories	Protein	Fat
290	28g	15g

- Prep Time: 12 minutes
- Cook Time: 8 minutes
- Serves: 4

Avocado Tuna Salad Lettuce Wraps:

Ingredients:

- 2 cans tuna, drained
- 1 avocado, mashed
- 1/4 cup red onion, finely chopped
- 1/4 cup celery, finely chopped
- Lettuce leaves for wrapping

Instructions:

1. In a bowl, combine tuna, mashed avocado, red onion, and celery.

2. Spoon the mixture onto lettuce leaves and wrap.

Nutrition approx.

Calories	Protein	Fat
230	25g	12g

- Prep Time: 10 minutes
- Serves: 2

Mediterranean Grilled Sardines:

Ingredients:
- 8 fresh sardines, cleaned
- 2 tbsp olive oil
- 2 cloves garlic, minced
- 1 tsp dried oregano
- Lemon wedges for serving

Instructions:

1. Preheat the grill.

2. Rub sardines with olive oil, minced garlic, and oregano.

3. Grill until cooked, about 3-4 minutes per side. Serve with lemon wedges.

Nutrition approx.

Calories	Protein	Fat
270	22g	18g

- Prep Time: 15 minutes
- Cook Time:8 minutes
- Serves: 4

Thai Basil Shrimp Stir-Fry:

Ingredients:
- 1 lb shrimp, peeled and deveined
- 2 cups broccoli florets
- 1 bell pepper, sliced
- 2 tbsp soy sauce
- 1 tbsp fish sauce
- Fresh basil leaves for garnish

Instructions:
1. In a wok, stir-fry shrimp, broccoli, and bell pepper.

2. Add soy sauce and fish sauce. Cook until shrimp is pink.

3. Garnish with fresh basil leaves before serving.

Nutrition approx.

Calories	Protein	Fat
280	25g	10g

- Prep Time: 15 minutes
- Cook Time:10 minutes
- Serves: 3

Lemon Herb Baked Cod:

Ingredients:
- 4 cod filets
- 3 tbsp lemon juice
- 2 tbsp olive oil
- 1 tsp dried thyme
- Salt and pepper to taste

Instructions:
1. Preheat the oven.
2. Place cod filets on a baking sheet.
3. Mix lemon juice, olive oil, thyme, salt, and pepper. Brush over cod.
4. Bake until the fish is opaque and flakes easily.

Nutrition approx.

Calories	Protein	Fat

250	30g	12g

- Prep Time: 10 minutes
- Cook Time: 15 minutes
- Serves: 4

Coconut Lime Shrimp Skewers:

Ingredients:
- 1 lb shrimp, peeled and deveined
- 1/2 cup coconut milk
- Zest and juice of 2 limes
- 2 tbsp cilantro, chopped
- Wooden skewers, soaked in water

Instructions:
1. In a bowl, marinate shrimp in coconut milk, lime zest, lime juice, and cilantro.
2. Thread shrimp onto skewers and grill until cooked.

Nutrition approx.

Calories	Protein	Fat
230	20g	14g

- Prep Time: 20 minutes
- Cook Time: 8 minutes
- Serves: 3

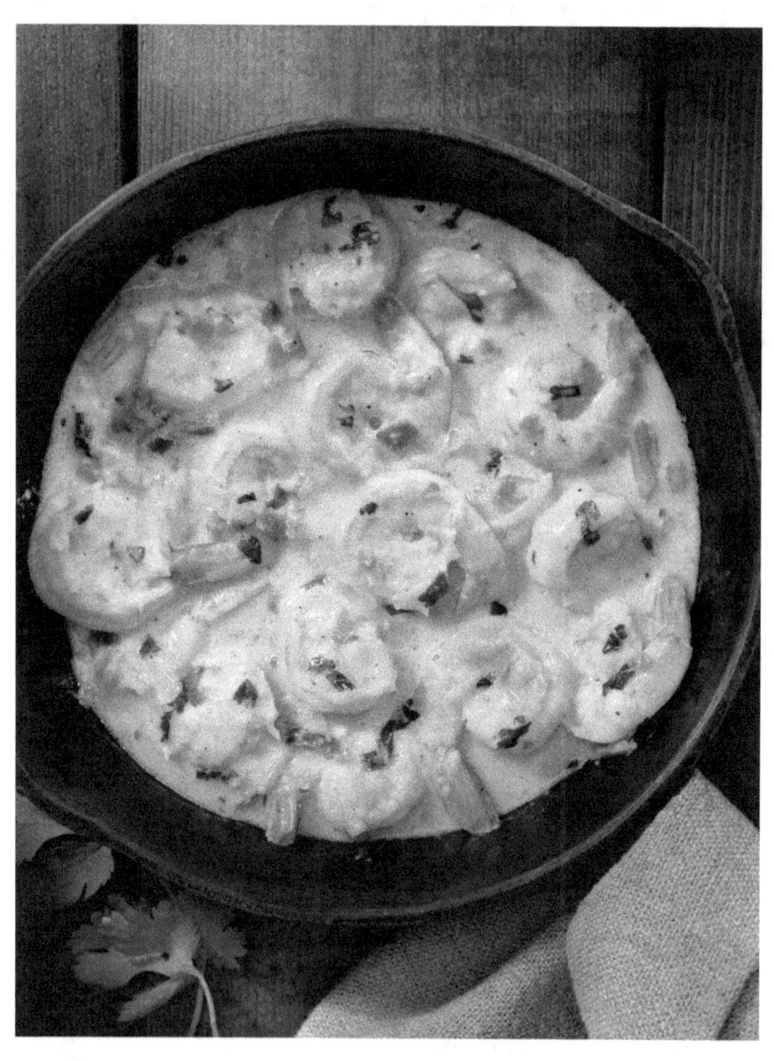

CHAPTER 5:

VEGETABLES RECIPES

Roasted Brussels Sprouts with Balsamic Glaze:

Ingredients:
- 1 lb Brussels sprouts, halved
- 2 tbsp olive oil
- Salt and pepper to taste
- 2 tbsp balsamic glaze

Instructions:
1. Preheat the oven.
2. Toss Brussels sprouts in olive oil, salt, and pepper.
3. Roast until crispy and browned.
4. Drizzle with balsamic glaze before serving.

Nutrition approx.

Calories	Protein	Fat
120	4g	7g

- Prep Time: 10 minutes
- Cook Time: 20 minutes
- Serves: 4

Zucchini Noodles with Pesto:

Ingredients:
- 4 medium zucchinis, spiralized
- 1/2 cup cherry tomatoes, halved
- 1/4 cup pine nuts
- 1/2 cup fresh basil
- 2 tbsp grated Parmesan
- 2 tbsp olive oil

Instructions:
1. Spiralize zucchini into noodles.
2. In a pan, sauté zucchini noodles, cherry tomatoes, and pine nuts in olive oil.
3. Toss with fresh basil and Parmesan.

Nutrition approx.

Calories	Protein	Fat
150	5g	10g

- Prep Time: 15 minutes
- Cook Time: 5 minutes
- Serves: 2

Spaghetti Squash Primavera:

Ingredients:
- 1 medium spaghetti squash
- 1 cup cherry tomatoes, halved
- 1 bell pepper, thinly sliced
- 1 zucchini, diced
- 2 tbsp olive oil
- 1 tsp Italian seasoning

Instructions:

1. Roast spaghetti squash until fork-tender.

2. In a pan, sauté cherry tomatoes, bell pepper, and zucchini in olive oil.

3. Scrape the spaghetti squash into the pan, add Italian seasoning, and toss.

Nutrition approx.

Calories	Protein	Fat
180	3g	8g

- Prep Time: 20 minutes
- Cook Time: 40 minutes
- Serves: 4

Stir-Fried Broccoli and Snow Peas:

Ingredients:

- 2 cups broccoli florets
- 1 cup snow peas, trimmed
- 2 tbsp soy sauce
- 1 tbsp sesame oil
- 1 tsp ginger, minced

Instructions:

1. In a wok, stir-fry broccoli and snow peas in sesame oil.

2. Add soy sauce and ginger, cook until vegetables are tender-crisp.

Nutrition approx.

Calories	Protein	Fat
90	4g	5g

- Prep Time: 10 minutes
- Cook Time: 8 minutes
- Serves: 3

Grilled Eggplant with Tomato and Feta:

Ingredients:
- 2 large eggplants, sliced
- 1 cup cherry tomatoes, halved
- 1/2 cup crumbled feta cheese
- 2 tbsp balsamic glaze
- Fresh basil for garnish

Instructions:

1. Grill eggplant slices until tender.
2. Top with cherry tomatoes, feta, and   drizzle with balsamic glaze.
3. Garnish with fresh basil.

Nutrition approx.

Calories	Protein	Fat
160	6g	8g

- Prep Time: 15 minutes
- Cook Time: 10 minutes
- Serves: 4

Quinoa Stuffed Bell Peppers:

Ingredients:

- 4 bell peppers, halved
- 1 cup quinoa, cooked
- 1 can black beans, drained and rinsed
- 1 cup corn kernels
- 1 cup diced tomatoes
- 1 tsp cumin
- Salt and pepper to taste

Instructions:

1. Preheat the oven.

2. Mix cooked quinoa, black beans, corn, diced tomatoes, cumin, salt, and pepper.

3. Stuff bell peppers with the quinoa mixture and bake until peppers are tender.

Nutrition approx.

Calories	Protein	Fat
200	8g	2g

- Prep Time: 20 minutes
- Cook Time: 25 minutes
- Serves: 4

Cauliflower Fried Rice:

Ingredients:
- 1 head cauliflower, grated
- 1 cup mixed vegetables (peas, carrots, corn)
- 2 eggs, beaten
- 2 tbsp soy sauce
- 1 tbsp sesame oil
- Green onions for garnish

Instructions:

1. In a pan, sauté cauliflower and mixed vegetables until tender.

2. Push vegetables to one side and scramble eggs on the other side.

3. Mix everything together, add soy sauce, and drizzle with sesame oil.

4. Garnish with chopped green onions.

Nutrition approx.

Calories	Protein	Fat
180	10g	8g

- Prep Time: 15 minutes
- Cook Time: 10 minutes
- Serves: 3

Spinach and Mushroom Quiche:

Ingredients:
- 1 pie crust
- 2 cups spinach, chopped
- 1 cup mushrooms, sliced
- 4 eggs
- 1 cup milk
- 1 cup shredded cheese
- Salt and pepper to taste

Instructions:
1. Preheat the oven.
2. Sauté spinach and mushrooms until cooked.
3. In a bowl, whisk eggs, milk, cheese, salt, and pepper.

4. Pour egg mixture into the pie crust, add sautéed vegetables, and bake until set.

Nutrition approx.

Calories	Protein	Fat
220	12g	14g

- Prep Time: 20 minutes
- Cook Time: 30 minutes
- Serves: 6

Ratatouille:

Ingredients:
- 1 eggplant, sliced
- 1 zucchini, sliced
- 1 yellow squash, sliced
- 1 bell pepper, sliced
- 1 onion, sliced
- 2 cups diced tomatoes
- 2 cloves garlic, minced
- 2 tbsp olive oil
- 1 tsp dried thyme
- Salt and pepper to taste

Instructions:
1. Preheat the oven.
2. Arrange sliced vegetables in a baking dish.

3. Mix diced tomatoes, minced garlic, olive oil, thyme, salt, and pepper. Pour over the vegetables.

4. Bake until vegetables are tender.

Nutrition approx.

Calories	Protein	Fat
180	5g	10g

- Prep Time:25 minutes
- Cook Time: 40 minutes
- Serves: 4

Broccoli and Cheddar Stuffed Sweet Potatoes:

Ingredients:
- 4 medium sweet potatoes, baked
- 2 cups broccoli florets, steamed
- 1 cup shredded cheddar cheese
- 1/2 cup Greek yogurt
- Salt and pepper to taste

Instructions:

1. Slice baked sweet potatoes in half.

2. Mash the insides and top with steamed broccoli, cheddar cheese, Greek yogurt, salt, and pepper.

Nutrition approx.

Calories	Protein	Fat
250	10g	8g

- Prep Time:15 minutes
- Cook Time: 45 minutes (including baking sweet potatoes)
- Serves: 4

Cabbage and Carrot Slaw:

Ingredients:
- 4 cups shredded cabbage
- 2 carrots, grated
- 1/4 cup Greek yogurt
- 1 tbsp Dijon mustard
- 1 tbsp apple cider vinegar
- Salt and pepper to taste

Instructions:

1. In a large bowl, combine shredded cabbage and grated carrots.

2. In a separate bowl, mix Greek yogurt, Dijon mustard, apple cider vinegar, salt, and pepper.

3. Pour the dressing over the cabbage and carrots, toss until well coated.

Nutrition approx.

Calories	Protein	Fat
120	3g	5g

- Prep Time: 15 minutes
- Serves: 4

Roasted Cauliflower Steak:

Ingredients:

- 1 large cauliflower head, sliced into steaks
- 2 tbsp olive oil
- 1 tsp smoked paprika
- 1/2 tsp garlic powder
- Salt and pepper to taste

Instructions:

1. Preheat the oven.
2. Place cauliflower steaks on a baking sheet.
3. Mix olive oil, smoked paprika, garlic powder, salt, and pepper. Brush over cauliflower.
4. Roast until golden brown and tender.

Nutrition approx.

Calories	Protein	Fat
100	5g	7g

- Prep Time: 10 minutes

- Cook Time: 25 minutes
- Serves: 2

Butternut Squash and Kale Salad:

Ingredients:
- 2 cups butternut squash, diced and roasted
- 3 cups kale, chopped
- 1/4 cup dried cranberries
- 1/4 cup feta cheese, crumbled
- 2 tbsp balsamic vinaigrette

Instructions:
1. Roast diced butternut squash until tender.
2. In a large bowl, combine roasted squash, chopped kale, dried cranberries, and feta cheese.
3. Drizzle with balsamic vinaigrette and toss.

Nutrition approx.

Calories	Protein	Fat
150	5g	8g

- Prep Time: 20 minutes
- Cook Time: 20 minutes
- Serves: 3

Asparagus and Mushroom Stir-Fry:

Ingredients:
- 1 lb asparagus, trimmed and cut into pieces
- 1 cup mushrooms, sliced
- 1 tbsp sesame oil
- 2 tbsp soy sauce
- 1 tsp honey
- 1 tsp ginger, minced

Instructions:

1. In a wok, stir-fry asparagus and mushrooms in sesame oil.

2. Mix soy sauce, honey, and minced ginger. Add to the wok and cook until vegetables are tender.

Nutrition approx.

Calories	Protein	Fat
90	5g	5g

- Prep Time: 15 minutes
- Cook Time: 10 minutes
- Serves: 3

Spinach and Artichoke Stuffed Portobello Mushrooms:

Ingredients:

- 4 large portobello mushrooms
- 2 cups fresh spinach
- 1 cup artichoke hearts, chopped
- 1/2 cup feta cheese, crumbled
- 2 tbsp olive oil

Instructions:
1. Preheat the oven.
2. Remove the stems from portobello mushrooms.
3. Sauté spinach and artichoke hearts in olive oil until wilted.
4. Stuff the portobello mushrooms with the spinach and artichoke mixture, top with feta cheese.
5. Bake until mushrooms are tender.

Nutrition approx.

Calories	Protein	Fat
160	7g	10g

-Prep Time:20 minutes
-Cook Time: 20 minutes
-Serves: 4

Mediterranean Chickpea Salad:

Ingredients:
- 2 cans chickpeas, drained and rinsed
- 1 cucumber, diced

- 1 cup cherry tomatoes, halved
- 1/2 cup red onion, finely chopped
- 1/4 cup Kalamata olives, sliced
- 2 tbsp olive oil
- 1 tbsp red wine vinegar
- 1 tsp dried oregano
- Salt and pepper to taste

Instructions:

1. In a large bowl, combine chickpeas, cucumber, cherry tomatoes, red onion, and olives.

2. In a small bowl, whisk together olive oil, red wine vinegar, dried oregano, salt, and pepper.

3. Pour the dressing over the salad and toss until well combined.

Nutrition approx.

Calories	Protein	Fat
220	8g	10g

- Prep Time: 15 minutes
- Serves: 4

Sweet Potato and Black Bean Chili:

Ingredients:

- 2 sweet potatoes, peeled and diced
- 1 can black beans, drained and rinsed

- 1 can diced tomatoes
- 1 onion, diced
- 2 cloves garlic, minced
- 2 tsp chili powder
- 1 tsp cumin
- Salt and pepper to taste

Instructions:

1. In a pot, sauté onions and garlic until fragrant.

2. Add sweet potatoes, black beans, diced tomatoes, chili powder, cumin, salt, and pepper.

3. Simmer until sweet potatoes are tender.

Nutrition approx.

Calories	Protein	Fat
180	5g	1g

- Prep Time: 20 minutes
- Cook Time: 25 minutes
- Serves: 4

Caprese Stuffed Avocados:

Ingredients:
- 2 avocados, halved and pitted
- 1 cup cherry tomatoes, halved
- 1/2 cup fresh mozzarella balls, halved
- Fresh basil leaves, torn

- Balsamic glaze for drizzling
- Salt and pepper to taste

Instructions:

1. Scoop out some flesh from each avocado half to create a larger well.

2. In a bowl, mix cherry tomatoes, fresh mozzarella, and torn basil.

3. Spoon the mixture into the avocado wells.

4. Drizzle with balsamic glaze and season with salt and pepper.

Nutrition approx.

Calories	Protein	Fat
250	6g	20g

- Prep Time: 15 minutes
- Serves: 2

Eggplant Parmesan:

Ingredients:

- 1 large eggplant, sliced
- 1 cup marinara sauce
- 1 cup mozzarella cheese, shredded
- 1/2 cup Parmesan cheese, grated
- 1/4 cup fresh basil, chopped
- 2 tbsp olive oil

- Salt and pepper to taste

Instructions:
1. Preheat the oven.
2. Brush eggplant slices with olive oil and season with salt and pepper.
3. In a baking dish, layer eggplant, marinara sauce, mozzarella, and Parmesan.
4. Repeat layers and bake until bubbly and golden.

Nutrition approx.

Calories	Protein	Fat
220	10g	15g

- Prep Time: 25 minutes
- Cook Time: 35 minutes
- Serves: 4

Cucumber and Avocado Sushi Rolls:

Ingredients:
- 2 cups cauliflower rice, cooked
- 4 nori sheets
- 1 cucumber, julienned
- 1 avocado, sliced
- Soy sauce for dipping
- Pickled ginger and wasabi for serving

Instructions:

1. Place a nori sheet on a bamboo sushi mat.

2. Spread cauliflower rice evenly on the nori sheet.

3. Add julienned cucumber and sliced avocado.

4. Roll tightly, slice into rolls, and serve with soy sauce, pickled ginger, and wasabi.

Nutrition approx.

Calories	Protein	Fat
180	5g	10g

- Prep Time: 30 minutes
- Serves: 2

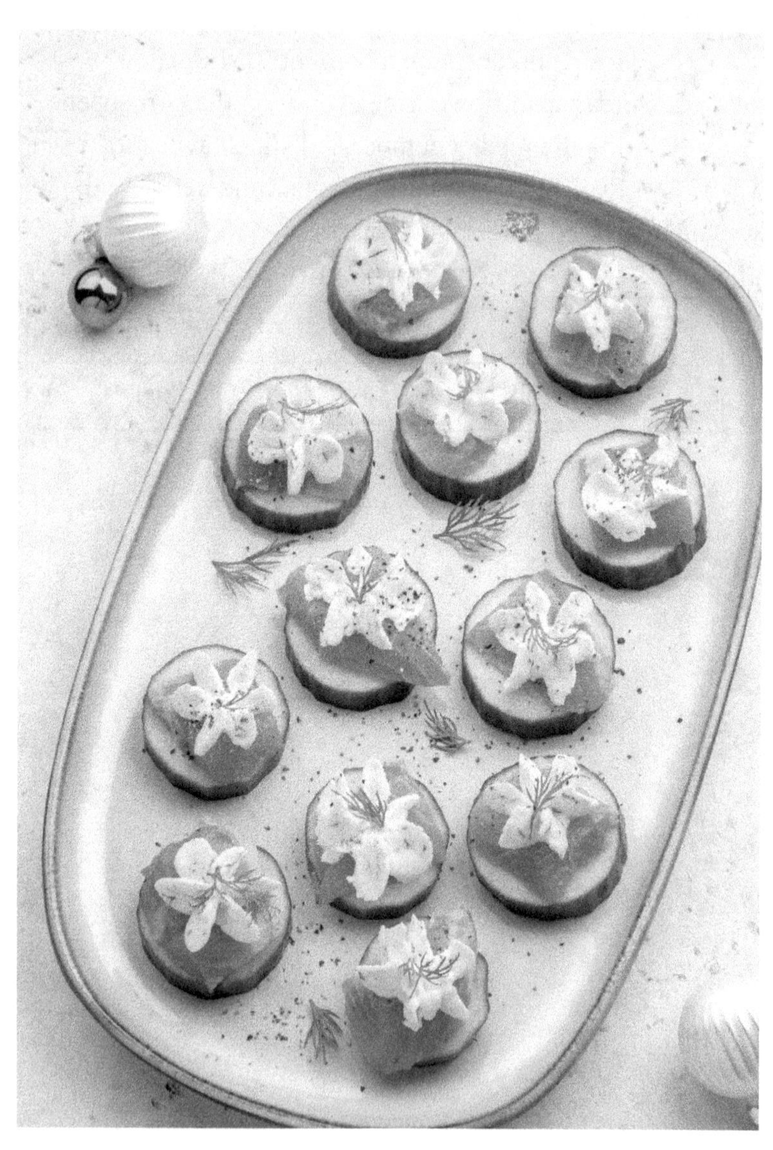

CHAPTER 6:

APPETIZER AND SNACK RECIPES

Guacamole Stuffed Cucumber Cups:

Ingredients:
- 2 cucumbers, sliced into rounds
- 2 avocados, mashed
- 1 tomato, diced
- 1/4 cup red onion, finely chopped
- 1 clove garlic, minced
- 1 lime, juiced
- Salt and pepper to taste
- Fresh cilantro for garnish

Instructions:
1. Scoop out a small well in each cucumber round.
2. In a bowl, mix mashed avocados, diced tomato, red onion, minced garlic, lime juice, salt, and pepper.
3. Spoon the guacamole into the cucumber cups.
4. Garnish with fresh cilantro.

Nutrition approx.

Calories	Protein	Fat
120	2g	10g

- Prep Time: 15 minutes
- Serves: 4

Smoked Salmon Cucumber Bites:

Ingredients:
- 1 cucumber, sliced into rounds
- 4 oz smoked salmon
- 1/4 cup cream cheese
- Fresh dill for garnish
- Capers for topping (optional)

Instructions:
1. Place a small dollop of cream cheese on each cucumber round.
2. Top with smoked salmon.
3. Garnish with fresh dill and capers if desired.

Nutrition approx.

Calories	Protein	Fat
90	8g	5g

- Prep Time:10 minutes
- Serves: 4

Greek Yogurt and Berry Parfait:

Ingredients:
  - 1 cup Greek yogurt
  - 1/2 cup mixed berries (strawberries,   blueberries, raspberries)
  - 2 tbsp honey
  - 2 tbsp granola

Instructions:
1. In a glass, layer Greek yogurt, mixed berries, and honey.
2. Repeat the layers.
3. Top with granola.

Nutrition approx.

Calories	Protein	Fat
180	15g	5g

- Prep Time: 10 minutes
- Serves: 2

Spicy Edamame:

Ingredients:

- 2 cups edamame, steamed
- 1 tbsp sesame oil
- 1 tsp soy sauce
- 1/2 tsp chili flakes
- Sesame seeds for garnish

Instructions:

1. In a bowl, toss steamed edamame with sesame oil, soy sauce, and chili flakes.

2. Garnish with sesame seeds.

Nutrition approx.

Calories	Protein	Fat
160	14g	8g

- Prep Time: 5 minutes
- Serves: 2

Caprese Skewers:

Ingredients:
- Cherry tomatoes
- Fresh mozzarella balls
- Fresh basil leaves
- Balsamic glaze for drizzling

Instructions:

1. Thread a cherry tomato, a mozzarella ball, and a basil leaf onto small skewers.

2. Arrange on a serving platter.

3. Drizzle with balsamic glaze before serving.

Nutrition approx.

Calories	Protein	Fat
90	5g	6g

- Prep Time: 10 minutes
- Serves: 4

Almond Butter and Banana Bites:

Ingredients:
- 2 bananas, sliced
- 1/4 cup almond butter
- Chia seeds for topping

Instructions:

1. Spread almond butter on banana slices.

2. Sprinkle it with chia seeds.

Nutrition approx.

Calories	Protein	Fat
120	3g	7g

- Prep Time: 5 minutes

- Serves: 2

Spinach and Artichoke Dip:

Ingredients:
- 1 cup frozen chopped spinach, thawed and drained
- 1 can artichoke hearts, chopped
- 1 cup Greek yogurt
- 1/2 cup mayonnaise
- 1 cup shredded mozzarella cheese
- 1/4 cup grated Parmesan cheese
- 1 tsp garlic powder
- Salt and pepper to taste
- Whole-grain crackers or vegetable sticks for dipping

Instructions:
1. Preheat the oven.

2. In a bowl, mix together spinach, artichoke hearts, Greek yogurt, mayonnaise, mozzarella cheese, Parmesan cheese, garlic powder, salt, and pepper.

3. Transfer the mixture to a baking dish and bake until bubbly and golden.

4. Serve with whole-grain crackers or vegetable sticks.

Nutrition approx.

Calories	Protein	Fat
150	8g	10g

- Prep Time: 15 minutes
- Cook Time: 25 minutes
- Serves: 4

Roasted Red Pepper Hummus:

Ingredients:
- 1 can chickpeas, drained and rinsed
- 1/4 cup tahini
- 1/4 cup lemon juice
- 2 tbsp olive oil
- 1/2 cup roasted red peppers
- 1 clove garlic
- 1/2 tsp cumin
- Salt and pepper to taste
- Whole-grain pita bread or vegetable sticks for dipping

Instructions:

1. In a food processor, blend chickpeas, tahini, lemon juice, olive oil, roasted red peppers, garlic, cumin, salt, and pepper until smooth.

2. Adjust seasoning to taste.

3. Serve with whole-grain pita bread or vegetable sticks.

Nutrition approx.

Calories	Protein	Fat
120	4g	8g

- Prep Time: 10 minutes
- Serves: 4

Quinoa and Black Bean Stuffed Mini Peppers:

Ingredients:
- 12 mini bell peppers, halved and seeds removed
- 1 cup cooked quinoa
- 1 can black beans, drained and rinsed
- 1 cup corn kernels
- 1/2 cup cherry tomatoes, diced
- 1/4 cup fresh cilantro, chopped
- 1 tsp cumin
- Salt and pepper to taste

Instructions:
1. Preheat the oven.
2. In a bowl, mix together cooked quinoa, black beans, corn, cherry tomatoes, cilantro, cumin, salt, and pepper.
3. Stuff each mini pepper half with the quinoa mixture.
4. Bake until peppers are tender.

Calories	Protein	Fat
110	4g	2g

- Prep Time: 20 minutes
- Cook Time: 15 minutes
- Serves: 4

Deviled Eggs with Avocado:

Ingredients:
- 6 hard-boiled eggs, peeled and halved
- 1 ripe avocado, mashed
- 2 tbsp Greek yogurt
- 1 tsp Dijon mustard
- Salt and pepper to taste
- Paprika for garnish

Instructions:
1. Remove egg yolks and place them in a bowl.
2. Mash egg yolks with mashed avocado, Greek yogurt, Dijon mustard, salt, and pepper.
3. Spoon the mixture back into egg whites.
4. Garnish with a sprinkle of paprika.

Nutrition approx.

Calories	Protein	Fat

90	6g	7g

- Prep Time: 15 minutes
- Serves: 3

Greek Yogurt and Cucumber Dip:

Ingredients:
- 1 cup Greek yogurt
- 1 cucumber, finely diced
- 1 clove garlic, minced
- 1 tbsp fresh dill, chopped
- 1 tbsp lemon juice
- Salt and pepper to taste
- Whole-grain crackers or vegetable sticks for dipping

Instructions:

1. In a bowl, combine Greek yogurt, diced cucumber, minced garlic, dill, lemon juice, salt, and pepper.

2. Mix well and refrigerate for at least 30 minutes before serving.

3. Serve with whole-grain crackers or vegetable sticks.

Nutrition approx.

Calories	Protein	Fat
70	6g	3g

- Prep Time:10 minutes
- Serves: 4

Baked Sweet Potato Fries:

Ingredients:
- 2 sweet potatoes, cut into fries
- 1 tbsp olive oil
- 1 tsp paprika
- 1/2 tsp garlic powder
- 1/2 tsp cumin
- Salt and pepper to taste

Instructions:
1. Preheat the oven.
2. Toss sweet potato fries with olive oil, paprika, garlic powder, cumin, salt, and pepper.
3. Spread on a baking sheet and bake until golden and crispy.

Nutrition approx.

Calories	Protein	Fat
120	2g	4g

- Prep Time: 15 minutes
- Cook Time: 25 minutes
- Serves: 4

Greek Quinoa Salad Cups:

Ingredients:
- 1 cup cooked quinoa
- 1 cup cucumber, diced
- 1 cup cherry tomatoes, halved
- 1/2 cup Kalamata olives, sliced
- 1/4 cup feta cheese, crumbled
- 2 tbsp red onion, finely chopped
- 2 tbsp olive oil
- 1 tbsp red wine vinegar
- Salt and pepper to taste
- Mini phyllo cups for serving

Instructions:

1. In a bowl, combine quinoa, cucumber, cherry tomatoes, olives, feta cheese, red onion, olive oil, red wine vinegar, salt, and pepper.

2. Spoon the mixture into mini phyllo cups.

3. Serve immediately.

Nutrition approx.

Calories	Protein	Fat
120	4g	6g

- Prep Time: 15 minutes
- Serves: 4

Turkey and Avocado Lettuce Wraps:

Ingredients:

- 8 large lettuce leaves (such as iceberg or Romaine)
- 1/2 lb deli turkey slices
- 1 avocado, sliced
- 1/2 cup cherry tomatoes, diced
- 1/4 cup red onion, thinly sliced
- Mustard or Greek yogurt dressing for drizzling

Instructions:

1. Lay out lettuce leaves.
2. Fill each leaf with turkey slices, avocado slices, cherry tomatoes, and red onion.
3. Drizzle with mustard or Greek yogurt dressing.

Nutrition approx.

Calories	Protein	Fat
130	12g	7g

- Prep Time: 10 minutes
- Serves: 4

Baked Zucchini Chips:

Ingredients:

- 2 zucchini, thinly sliced
- 1/4 cup grated Parmesan cheese

- 1/4 cup whole wheat breadcrumbs
- 1 tsp garlic powder
- 1/2 tsp dried oregano
- Olive oil spray

Instructions:

1. Preheat the oven.

2. In a bowl, mix Parmesan cheese, breadcrumbs, garlic powder, and dried oregano.

3. Dip zucchini slices in the mixture and place on a baking sheet.

4. Lightly spray with olive oil and bake until golden and crispy.

Nutrition approx.

Calories	Protein	Fat
80	5g	3g

- Prep Time: 15 minutes
- Cook Time: 20 minutes
- Serves: 4

Blueberry and Almond Yogurt Parfait:

Ingredients:

- 1 cup Greek yogurt
- 1/2 cup blueberries
- 2 tbsp almonds, chopped

- 1 tbsp honey
- 1/2 tsp vanilla extract

Instructions:

1. In a glass, layer Greek yogurt, blueberries, and chopped almonds.

2. Drizzle with honey and add a splash of vanilla extract.

3. Repeat the layers.

Nutrition approx.

Calories	Protein	Fat
180	15g	8g

- Prep Time: 10 minutes
- Serves:2

Stuffed Mushrooms with Spinach and Feta:

Ingredients:

- 12 large mushrooms, cleaned and stems removed
- 1 cup fresh spinach, chopped
- 1/2 cup feta cheese, crumbled
- 2 cloves garlic, minced
- 1 tbsp olive oil
- Salt and pepper to taste

Instructions:

1. Preheat the oven.

2. In a skillet, sauté spinach and garlic in olive oil until wilted.

3. Stuff each mushroom with the spinach mixture and top with feta cheese.

4. Bake until mushrooms are tender.

Nutrition approx.

Calories	Protein	Fat
90	5g	6g

- Prep Time: 20 minutes
- Cook Time: 15 minutes
- Serves: 4

Chia Pudding with Mixed Berries:

Ingredients:
- 3 tbsp chia seeds
- 1 cup almond milk
- 1/2 tsp vanilla extract
- 1 tbsp maple syrup
- 1/2 cup mixed berries (strawberries, blueberries, raspberries)

Instructions:

1. In a jar, mix chia seeds, almond milk, vanilla extract, and maple syrup.

2. Stir well and refrigerate overnight or until the mixture thickens.

3. Before serving, top with mixed berries.

Nutrition approx.

Calories	Protein	Fat
150	4g	7g

- Prep Time: 5 minutes (plus overnight refrigeration)
- Serves: 2

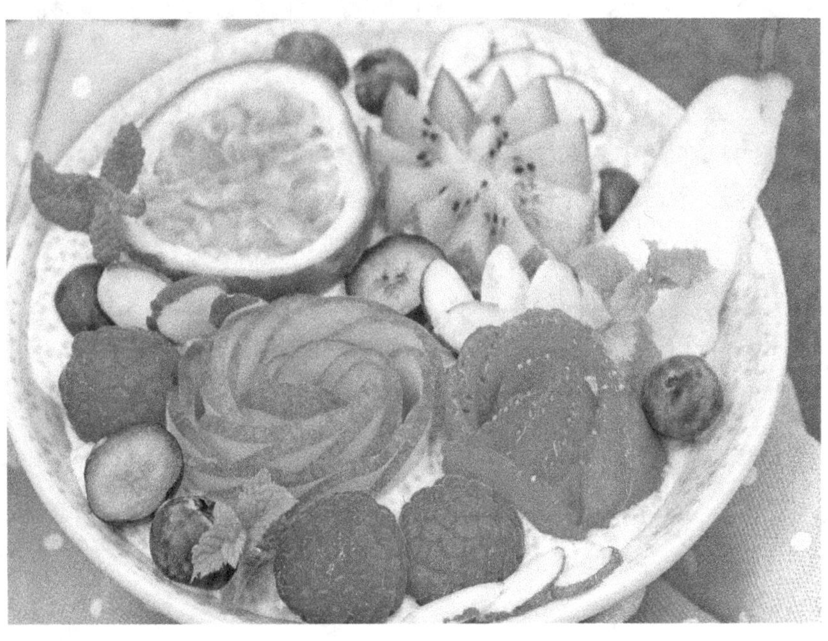

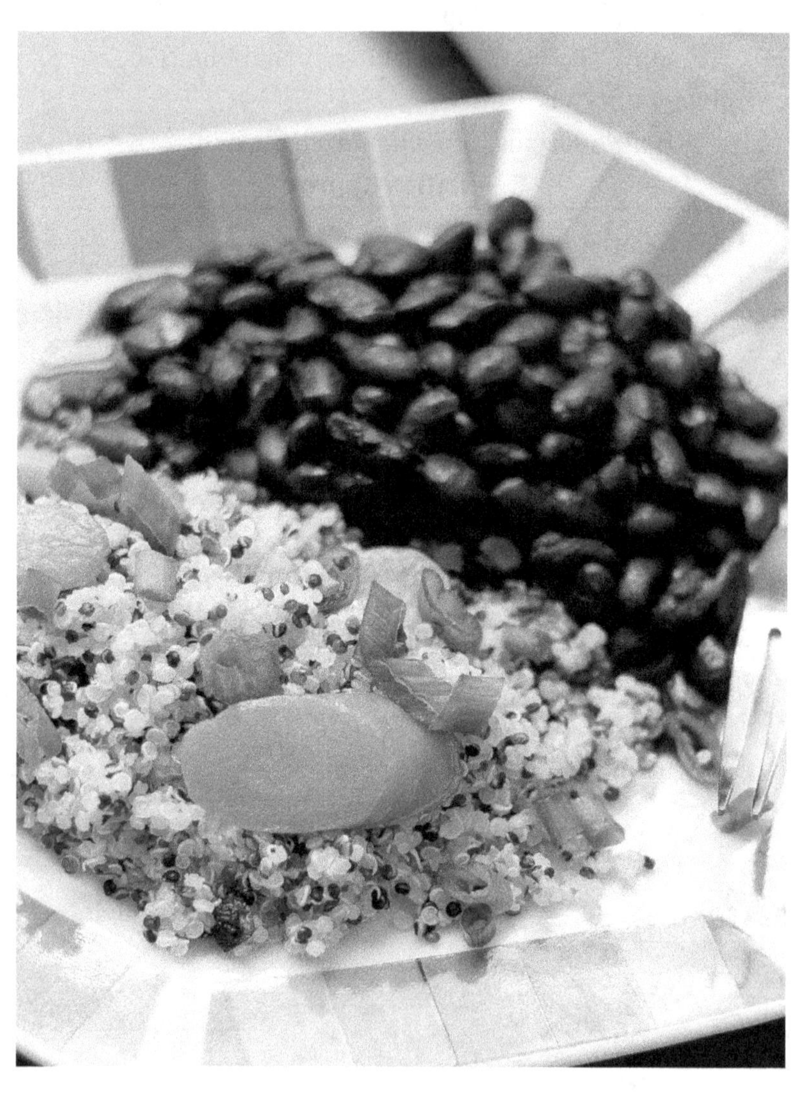

CHAPTER 7:

BEANS,PASTA & GRAINS RECIPES

Quinoa and Black Bean Bowl:

Ingredients:
- 1 cup cooked quinoa
- 1 can black beans, drained and rinsed
- 1 cup cherry tomatoes, halved
- 1/2 cup corn kernels
- 1/4 cup red onion, finely chopped
- 1/4 cup cilantro, chopped
- 2 tbsp lime juice
- 1 tbsp olive oil
- Salt and pepper to taste
- Avocado slices for garnish

Instructions:

1. In a bowl, combine quinoa, black beans, cherry tomatoes, corn, red onion, and cilantro.

2. In a separate bowl, whisk together lime juice, olive oil, salt, and pepper.

3. Pour the dressing over the quinoa mixture and toss gently.

4. Garnish with avocado slices before serving.

Nutrition approx.

Calories	Protein	Fat
300	10g	8g

- Prep Time: 15 minutes
- Serves: 2

Lentil and Vegetable Stew:

Ingredients:
- 1 cup lentils, rinsed
- 4 cups vegetable broth
- 1 onion, diced
- 2 carrots, sliced
- 2 celery stalks, chopped
- 2 cloves garlic, minced
- 1 can diced tomatoes
- 1 tsp cumin
- 1 tsp paprika
- Salt and pepper to taste
- Fresh parsley for garnish

Instructions:

1. In a pot, combine lentils, vegetable broth, onion, carrots, celery, garlic, diced tomatoes, cumin, paprika, salt, and pepper.

2. Bring to a boil, then simmer until lentils are tender.

3. Garnish with fresh parsley before serving.

Nutrition approx.

Calories	Protein	Fat
250	15g	2g

- Prep Time: 10 minutes
- Cook Time: 30 minutes
- Serves: 4

Chickpea and Spinach Curry:

Ingredients:
- 1 can chickpeas, drained and rinsed
- 1 onion, diced
- 2 cloves garlic, minced
- 1 can coconut milk
- 1 can diced tomatoes
- 2 cups fresh spinach
- 1 tbsp curry powder
- 1 tsp turmeric
- Salt and pepper to taste
- Brown rice for serving

Instructions:

1. In a pan, sauté onion and garlic until softened.

2. Add chickpeas, coconut milk, diced tomatoes, spinach, curry powder, turmeric, salt, and pepper.

3. Simmer until the curry thickens.

4. Serve over brown rice.

Nutrition approx.

Calories	Protein	Fat
350	12g	15g

- Prep Time: 15 minutes
- Cook Time: 25 minutes
- Serves: 3

Whole Wheat Pasta with Pesto and Cherry Tomatoes:

Ingredients:

- 8 oz whole wheat pasta
- 1 cup fresh basil leaves
- 1/2 cup Parmesan cheese, grated
- 1/4 cup pine nuts
- 2 cloves garlic
- 1/2 cup extra virgin olive oil
- Salt and pepper to taste
- Cherry tomatoes, halved, for topping

Instructions:
1. Cook pasta according to package instructions.
2. In a food processor, blend basil, Parmesan, pine nuts, garlic, olive oil, salt, and pepper to make pesto.
3. Toss cooked pasta with pesto and top with cherry tomatoes.

Nutrition approx.

Calories	Protein	Fat
400	12g	20g

- Prep Time: 20 minutes
- Cook Time: 10 minutes
- Serves: 4

Wild Rice Salad with Cranberries and Almonds:

Ingredients:
- 1 cup wild rice, cooked
- 1/2 cup dried cranberries
- 1/2 cup slivered almonds, toasted
- 1/4 cup green onions, sliced
- 2 tbsp olive oil
- 1 tbsp balsamic vinegar
- Salt and pepper to taste
- Feta cheese for garnish

Instructions:

1. In a bowl, combine cooked wild rice, cranberries, almonds, and green onions.

2. In a small bowl, whisk together olive oil, balsamic vinegar, salt, and pepper.

3. Pour the dressing over the rice mixture and toss.

4. Garnish with crumbled feta cheese.

Nutrition approx.

Calories	Protein	Fat
300	8g	15g

- Prep Time: 15 minutes
- Serves: 3

Black Bean and Corn Quesadillas:

Ingredients:

- 1 can black beans, drained and rinsed

- 1 cup corn kernels
- 1/2 cup red bell pepper, diced
- 1/4 cup red onion, finely chopped
- 1 tsp cumin
- 1/2 tsp chili powder
- 4 whole wheat tortillas
- 1 cup shredded cheese (cheddar or Mexican blend)

- Greek yogurt and salsa for serving

Instructions:

1. In a bowl, mix black beans, corn, red bell pepper, red onion, cumin, and chili powder.

2. Place a tortilla on a skillet, add a portion of the bean mixture, and sprinkle with cheese.

3. Top with another tortilla and cook until cheese is melted.

4. Repeat for remaining tortillas.

5. Serve with Greek yogurt and salsa.

Nutrition approx.

Calories	Protein	Fat
350	15g	10g

- Prep Time: 20 minutes
- Cook Time: 10 minutes
- Serves: 2a

Spaghetti Squash with Tomato Basil Sauce:

Ingredients:

- 1 medium-sized spaghetti squash
- 2 cups cherry tomatoes, halved
- 2 cloves garlic, minced
- 1/4 cup fresh basil, chopped

- 2 tbsp olive oil
- Salt and pepper to taste
- Grated Parmesan cheese for topping

Instructions:
1. Preheat the oven.

2. Cut the spaghetti squash in half, scoop out the seeds, and roast until tender.

3. In a skillet, sauté cherry tomatoes and garlic in olive oil until tomatoes are soft.

4. Scrape the spaghetti squash into strands, mix with the tomato sauce, and top with fresh basil and Parmesan.

Nutrition approx.

Calories	Protein	Fat
250	5g	12g

- Prep Time: 15 minutes
- Cook Time: 40 minutes
- Serves: 2

Chickpea and Vegetable Stir-Fry:

Ingredients:
- 1 can chickpeas, drained and rinsed
- 2 cups broccoli florets
- 1 red bell pepper, sliced
- 1 carrot, julienned

- 1 cup snap peas
- 2 tbsp soy sauce
- 1 tbsp sesame oil
- 1 tsp ginger, minced
- 2 cloves garlic, minced
- Brown rice for serving

Instructions:

1. In a wok or skillet, stir-fry chickpeas, broccoli, red bell pepper, carrot, and snap peas in sesame oil.

2. Add soy sauce, ginger, and garlic. Stir until vegetables are tender.

3. Serve over brown rice.

Nutrition approx.

Calories	Protein	Fat
300	12g	10g

- Prep Time:15 minutes
- Cook Time: 10 minutes
- Serves: 3

Pesto and Sun-Dried Tomato Farro Salad:

Ingredients:
- 1 cup farro, cooked
- 1/4 cup pesto sauce

- 1/4 cup sun-dried tomatoes, chopped
- 1/4 cup Kalamata olives, sliced
- 1/4 cup feta cheese, crumbled
- 2 tbsp pine nuts, toasted
- Fresh basil for garnish

Instructions:

1. In a bowl, combine cooked farro, pesto sauce, sun-dried tomatoes, olives, feta cheese, and pine nuts.

2. Toss until well mixed.

3. Garnish with fresh basil before serving.

Nutrition approx.

Calories	Protein	Fat
280	8g	12g

- Prep Time: 20 minutes
- Serves: 2

Black-Eyed Pea and Vegetable Soup:

Ingredients:

- 1 cup black-eyed peas, soaked and cooked
- 4 cups vegetable broth
- 1 onion, diced
- 2 carrots, sliced
- 2 celery stalks, chopped
- 1 zucchini, diced

- 1 can diced tomatoes
- 1 tsp thyme
- 1 tsp rosemary
- Salt and pepper to taste

Instructions:

1. In a pot, combine black-eyed peas, vegetable broth, onion, carrots, celery, zucchini, diced tomatoes, thyme, rosemary, salt, and pepper.

2. Simmer until vegetables are tender.

3. Adjust seasoning if needed before serving.

Nutrition approx.

Calories	Protein	Fat
200	10g	1g

- Prep Time: 15 minutes
- Cook Time: 30 minutes
- Serves: 4

Spinach and Mushroom Stuffed Bell Peppers:

Ingredients:
- 4 bell peppers, halved and seeds removed
- 2 cups quinoa, cooked
- 1 cup spinach, chopped
- 1 cup mushrooms, diced

- 1 onion, finely chopped
- 2 cloves garlic, minced
- 1 tsp Italian seasoning
- 1/2 cup marinara sauce
- 1/2 cup mozzarella cheese, shredded

Instructions:

1. Preheat the oven.

2. In a skillet, sauté spinach, mushrooms, onion, and garlic until softened.

3. In a bowl, mix the cooked quinoa, sautéed vegetables, Italian seasoning, and marinara sauce.

4. Stuff each bell pepper half with the quinoa mixture and top with shredded mozzarella.

5. Bake until peppers are tender.

Nutrition approx.

Calories	Protein	Fat
320	12g	8g

- Prep Time: 20 minutes
- Cook Time: 25 minutes
- Serves: 4

Pasta e Fagioli:

Ingredients:

- 1 cup small pasta (such as ditalini)

- 1 can cannellini beans, drained and rinsed
- 2 cups vegetable broth
- 1 onion, diced
- 2 carrots, sliced
- 2 celery stalks, chopped
- 2 cloves garlic, minced
- 1 can diced tomatoes
- 1 tsp oregano
- 1 tsp basil
- Salt and pepper to taste

Instructions:

1. Cook pasta according to package instructions.

2. In a pot, combine cooked pasta, cannellini beans, vegetable broth, onion, carrots, celery, garlic, diced tomatoes, oregano, basil, salt, and pepper.

3. Simmer until vegetables are tender.

4. Adjust seasoning if needed before serving.

Nutrition approx.

Calories	Protein	Fat
250	10g	2g

- Prep Time: 15 minutes
- Cook Time: 20 minutes
- Serves: 3

Brown Rice and Black Bean Burrito Bowl:

Ingredients:
- 1 cup brown rice, cooked
- 1 can black beans, drained and rinsed
- 1 cup corn kernels
- 1 cup cherry tomatoes, diced
- 1/2 cup red onion, finely chopped
- 1/4 cup fresh cilantro, chopped
- 1 lime, juiced
- 1 tsp cumin
- Salt and pepper to taste
- Avocado slices for garnish

Instructions:

1. In a bowl, combine cooked brown rice, black beans, corn, cherry tomatoes, red onion, and cilantro.

2. Drizzle with lime juice, sprinkle with cumin, salt, and pepper.

3. Toss gently and garnish with avocado slices before serving.

Nutrition approx.

Calories	Protein	Fat
300	10g	5g

- Prep Time: 20 minutes

- Serves: 2

Chickpea and Avocado Salad:

Ingredients:
  - 1 can chickpeas, drained and rinsed
  - 1 avocado, diced
  - 1 cup cucumber, diced
  - 1/4 cup red onion, finely chopped
  - 2 tbsp fresh parsley, chopped
  - 2 tbsp olive oil
  - 1 tbsp red wine vinegar
  - Salt and pepper to taste

Instructions:

1. In a bowl, combine chickpeas, avocado, cucumber, red onion, and parsley.

2. In a small bowl, whisk together olive oil, red wine vinegar, salt, and pepper.

3. Drizzle the dressing over the salad and toss gently.

Nutrition approx.

Calories	Protein	Fat
250	8g	15g

- Prep Time: 15 minutes
- Serves: 2

Quinoa and Vegetable Stuffed Bell Peppers:

Ingredients:
- 4 bell peppers, halved and seeds removed
- 1 cup quinoa, cooked
- 1 cup black beans, cooked
- 1 cup corn kernels
- 1 cup cherry tomatoes, diced
- 1/2 cup red onion, finely chopped
- 1/4 cup fresh cilantro, chopped
- 1 tsp cumin
- Salt and pepper to taste
- Salsa for topping

Instructions:
1. Preheat the oven.
2. In a bowl, mix cooked quinoa, black beans, corn, cherry tomatoes, red onion, cilantro, cumin, salt, and pepper.
3. Stuff each bell pepper half with the quinoa mixture.
4. Bake until peppers are tender.
5. Top with salsa before serving.

Nutrition approx.

Calories	Protein	Fat
320	12g	6g

- Prep Time: 20 minutes
- Cook Time: 25 minutes
- Serves: 4

Whole Wheat Spaghetti with Lentil Bolognese:

Ingredients:
- 8 oz whole wheat spaghetti
- 1 cup green lentils, cooked
- 1 can diced tomatoes
- 1 onion, diced
- 2 carrots, grated
- 2 cloves garlic, minced
- 2 tbsp tomato paste
- 1 tsp dried oregano
- 1 tsp dried basil
- Salt and pepper to taste
- Fresh parsley for garnish

Instructions:
1. Cook whole wheat spaghetti according to package instructions.

2. In a skillet, sauté onion, garlic, and carrots until softened.

3. Add cooked lentils, diced tomatoes, tomato paste, oregano, basil, salt, and pepper.

4. Simmer until the sauce thickens.

5. Serve over whole wheat spaghetti and garnish with fresh parsley.

Nutrition approx.

Calories	Protein	Fat
350	15g	5g

- Prep Time: 15 minutes
- Cook Time: 30 minutes
- Serves: 3

Farro and Vegetable Stir-Fry:

Ingredients:
- 1 cup farro, cooked
- 1 cup broccoli florets
- 1 red bell pepper, sliced
- 1 cup snow peas
- 1 carrot, julienned
- 2 tbsp soy sauce
- 1 tbsp hoisin sauce
- 1 tsp sesame oil
- 1 tsp ginger, minced
- 2 cloves garlic, minced

Instructions:

1. In a wok or skillet, stir-fry cooked farro, broccoli, red bell pepper, snow peas, and carrot in sesame oil.

2. In a small bowl, mix soy sauce, hoisin sauce, ginger, and garlic.

3. Pour the sauce over the farro and vegetables. Stir until well coated.

4. Serve warm.

Nutrition approx.

Calories	Protein	Fat
280	10g	6g

- Prep Time: 20 minutes
- Serves: 2

Black Bean and Quinoa Stuffed Acorn Squash:

Ingredients:
- 2 acorn squash, halved and seeds removed
- 1 cup quinoa, cooked
- 1 can black beans, drained and rinsed
- 1 cup corn kernels
- 1/2 cup red onion, finely chopped
- 1/4 cup fresh cilantro, chopped
- 1 lime, juiced
- 1 tsp cumin
- Salt and pepper to taste

- Greek yogurt for topping

Instructions:
1. Preheat the oven.
2. Roast acorn squash halves until tender.
3. In a bowl, combine cooked quinoa, black beans, corn, red onion, cilantro, lime juice, cumin, salt, and pepper.
4. Stuff each acorn squash half with the quinoa mixture.
5. Top with a dollop of Greek yogurt before serving.

Nutrition approx.

Calories	Protein	Fat
320	12g	5g

- Prep Time: 25 minutes
- Cook Time: 40 minutes
- Serves: 4

CHAPTER 8:

APPETIZER AND SNACK RECIPES

Greek Yogurt and Berry Parfait:

Ingredients:
- 1 cup Greek yogurt
- 1/2 cup mixed berries (blueberries, strawberries, raspberries)
- 1 tbsp honey
- 2 tbsp granola

Instructions

1. In a glass, layer Greek yogurt, mixed berries, and granola.

2. Drizzle with honey.

3. Repeat the layers.

Nutrition approx.

Calories	Protein	Fat
150	10g	5g

- Prep Time: 5 minutes
- Serves: 1

Cucumber and Hummus Bites:

Ingredients:
- 1 cucumber, sliced
- 1/4 cup hummus
- Cherry tomatoes, halved
- Fresh parsley for garnish

Instructions:
1. Spread hummus on cucumber slices.
2. Top with cherry tomato halves.
3. Garnish with fresh parsley.

Nutrition approx.

Calories	Protein	Fat
50	2g	3g

- Prep Time: 10 minutes
- Serves: 2

Smoked Salmon and Avocado Roll-Ups:

Ingredients:
- 4 slices smoked salmon
- 1 avocado, sliced
- 1 tbsp cream cheese
- Fresh dill for garnish

Instructions:

1. Spread cream cheese on smoked salmon slices.
2. Place avocado slices on top.
3. Roll up and secure with a toothpick.
4. Garnish with fresh dill.

Nutrition approx.

Calories	Protein	Fat
120	8g	9g

- Prep Time: 15 minutes
- Serves: 2

Stuffed Cherry Tomatoes with Tuna Salad:

Ingredients:

- 12 cherry tomatoes, halved
- 1 can tuna, drained
- 2 tbsp Greek yogurt
- 1 tbsp Dijon mustard
- 1 celery stalk, finely chopped
- Salt and pepper to taste

Instructions:

1. In a bowl, mix tuna, Greek yogurt, Dijon mustard, celery, salt, and pepper.
2. Spoon the tuna salad into halved cherry tomatoes.

Nutrition approx.

Calories	Protein	Fat
100	15g	3g

- Prep Time: 10 minutes
- Serves: 4

Almond and Chia Energy Balls:

Ingredients:
- 1 cup almonds
- 1/4 cup chia seeds
- 1/4 cup honey
- 1/2 tsp vanilla extract
- Shredded coconut for rolling

Instructions:

1. In a food processor, blend almonds until finely ground.

2. Add chia seeds, honey, and vanilla extract. Pulse until combined.

3. Roll into small balls and coat with shredded coconut.

Nutrition approx.

Calories	Protein	Fat
80	3g	5g

- Prep Time: 15 minutes
- Serves: 12

Caprese Skewers with Balsamic Glaze:

Ingredients:
- Cherry tomatoes
- Mozzarella balls
- Fresh basil leaves
- Balsamic glaze

Instructions:
1. Thread a cherry tomato, a mozzarella ball, and a basil leaf onto each toothpick.
2. Drizzle with balsamic glaze before serving.

Nutrition approx.

Calories	Protein	Fat
70	5g	5g

- Prep Time: 10 minutes
- Serves: 6

Avocado and Salsa Dip with Veggie Sticks:

Ingredients:

- 2 avocados, mashed
- 1/2 cup salsa
- Carrot and cucumber sticks for dipping

Instructions:

1. Mix mashed avocados with salsa.
2. Serve with carrot and cucumber sticks.

Nutrition approx.

Calories	Protein	Fat
150	2g	12g

- Prep Time: 10 minutes
- Serves: 4

Egg Salad Lettuce Wraps:

Ingredients:

- 4 hard-boiled eggs, chopped
- 2 tbsp Greek yogurt
- 1 tsp Dijon mustard
- 1 celery stalk, finely chopped
- Lettuce leaves for wrapping

Instructions:

1. In a bowl, mix chopped eggs, Greek yogurt, Dijon mustard, and celery.
2. Spoon the egg salad on lettuce leaves.

Nutrition approx.

Calories	Protein	Fat
120	10g	8g

- Prep Time: 15 minutes
- Serves: 2

Quinoa and Black Bean Stuffed Mini Peppers:

Ingredients:
- 12 mini bell peppers, halved
- 1 cup quinoa, cooked
- 1/2 cup black beans, drained and rinsed
- 1/2 cup corn kernels
- 1/4 cup red onion, finely chopped
- 1/4 cup cilantro, chopped
- Lime wedges for garnish

Instructions:
1. Preheat the oven.
2. In a bowl, mix cooked quinoa, black beans, corn, red onion, and cilantro.
3. Stuff each mini pepper half with the quinoa mixture.
4. Bake until peppers are tender.
5. Garnish with lime wedges.

Nutrition approx.

Calories	Protein	Fat
90	4g	2g

- Prep Time: 20 minutes
- Cook Time: 15 minutes
- Serves: 4

Beet and Goat Cheese Crostini:

Ingredients:
- Baguette slices, toasted
- 1 cup roasted beets, sliced
- 1/2 cup goat cheese
- Honey for drizzling
- Fresh thyme for garnish

Instructions:
1. Spread goat cheese on toasted baguette slices.
2. Top with sliced roasted beets.
3. Drizzle with honey and garnish with fresh thyme.

Nutrition approx.

Calories	Protein	Fat
80	3g	4g

- Prep Time: 15 minutes

- Serves: 6

Spinach and Feta Stuffed Mushrooms:

Ingredients:
- 12 large mushrooms, stems removed
- 1 cup spinach, chopped
- 1/2 cup feta cheese, crumbled
- 2 cloves garlic, minced
- 1 tbsp olive oil
- Salt and pepper to taste

Instructions:
1. Preheat the oven.
2. In a skillet, sauté spinach and garlic in olive oil until wilted.
3. Mix sautéed spinach with crumbled feta.
4. Stuff mushrooms with the spinach and feta mixture.
5. Bake until mushrooms are tender.

Nutrition approx.

Calories	Protein	Fat
70	5g	4g

- Prep Time: 15 minutes
- Cook Time: 20 minutes
- Serves: 4

Zucchini and Carrot Fritters:

Ingredients:
- 1 zucchini, grated
- 1 carrot, grated
- 1/4 cup whole wheat flour
- 1 egg
- 1/4 cup feta cheese, crumbled
- 1/2 tsp cumin
- Salt and pepper to taste
- Greek yogurt for dipping

Instructions:

1. In a bowl, combine grated zucchini, grated carrot, whole wheat flour, egg, feta cheese, cumin, salt, and pepper.

2. Form into small patties and cook until golden brown.

3. Serve with a side of Greek yogurt for dipping.

Nutrition approx.

Calories	Protein	Fat
90	5g	5g

- Prep Time: 20 minutes
- Cook Time: 15 minutes
- Serves: 3

Mango Salsa with Cucumber Chips:

Ingredients:
- 1 mango, diced
- 1/2 red onion, finely chopped
- 1/2 red bell pepper, diced
- 1/4 cup fresh cilantro, chopped
- Juice of 1 lime
- Cucumber slices for dipping

Instructions:

1. In a bowl, combine diced mango, red onion, red bell pepper, cilantro, and lime juice.

2. Serve with cucumber slices for dipping.

Nutrition approx.

Calories	Protein	Fat
60	1g	1g

- Prep Time: 15 minutes
- Serves: 4

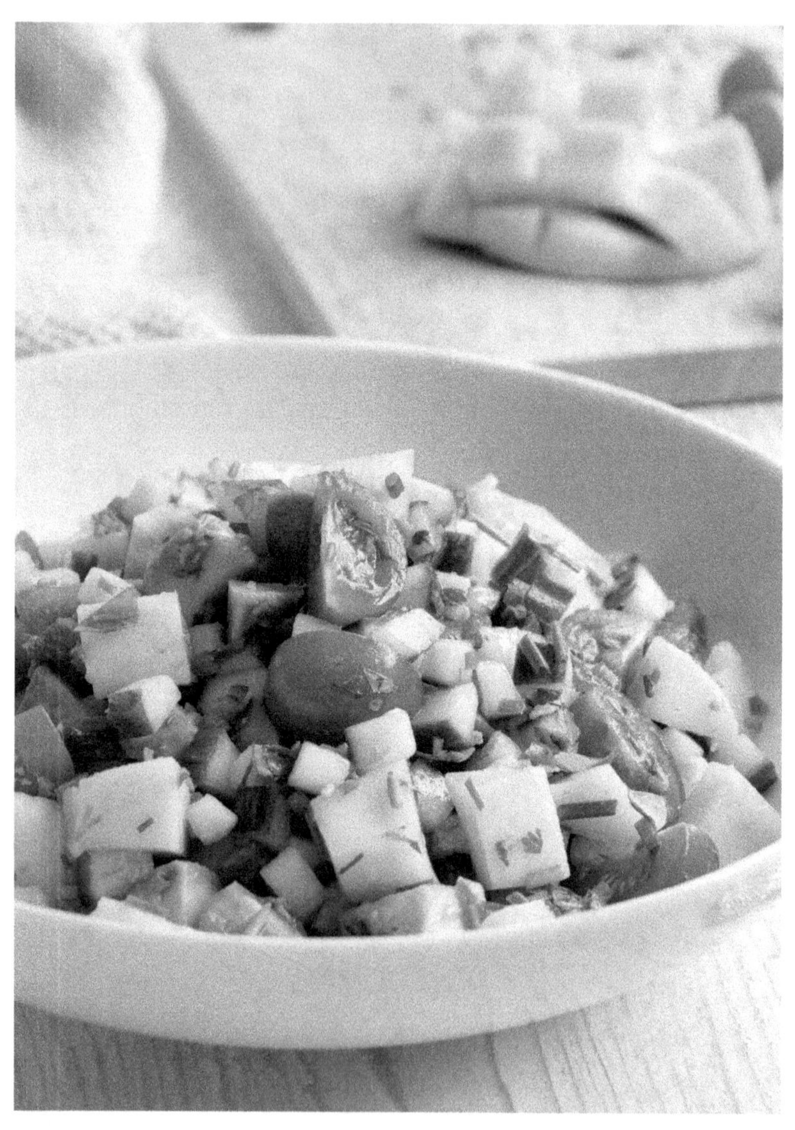

CHAPTER 9:

28-DAYS MEAL PLAN

DAY 1:

Breakfast (12 PM):
Avocado and Tomato Toast with Poached Egg

Ingredients:
  - 1 slice whole-grain bread
  - 1/2 avocado, mashed
  - 1 tomato, sliced
  - 1 poached egg
  - Salt and pepper to taste

Instructions:
  1. Toast the bread.
  2. Spread mashed avocado on the toast.
  3. Top with tomato slices and a poached egg.
  4. Season with salt and pepper.

Nutrition:
  - Approximately 300 calories, 15g protein, 15g fat.

Lunch (3 PM):
Quinoa Salad with Chickpeas, Cucumber, and Feta

- **Ingredients**:
  - 1 cup cooked quinoa
  - 1/2 cup chickpeas, drained and rinsed
  - 1 cucumber, diced
  - 1/4 cup feta cheese, crumbled
  - Olive oil and lemon dressing

- **Instructions**:
  1. In a bowl, combine quinoa, chickpeas, cucumber, and feta.
  2. Drizzle with olive oil and lemon dressing.

- **Nutrition**:
  - Approximately 350 calories, 12g protein, 15g fat.

Snack (6 PM)
Greek Yogurt with Berries and a Drizzle of Honey

-**Ingredients**:
  - 1 cup Greek yogurt
  - Mixed berries (strawberries, blueberries, raspberries)
  - 1 tablespoon honey

- **Instructions**:

1. In a bowl, mix Greek yogurt with berries.
2. Drizzle with honey.

- **Nutrition**:
  - Approximately 200 calories, 15g protein, 5g fat.

Dinner (8 PM):

Grilled Chicken Breast with Roasted Vegetables and Sweet Potato

-Ingredients:
  - 1 boneless, skinless chicken breast
  - Assorted vegetables (bell peppers, zucchini, cherry tomatoes)
  - 1 sweet potato, diced
  - Olive oil, garlic, and herbs for seasoning

- **Instructions:**
  1. Season the chicken breast with olive oil, garlic, and herbs, then grill.
  2. Roast vegetables and sweet potatoes in the oven.

- **Nutrition:**
  - Approximately 400 calories, 30g protein, 15g fat.

DAY 2:

Breakfast (12 PM):

Smoothie with Spinach, Banana, and Protein Powder

- **Ingredients:**
  - 1 cup spinach
  - 1 banana
  - 1 scoop protein powder
  - 1 cup almond milk

- **Instructions:**
  1. Blend all ingredients until smooth.

- **Nutrition:**
  - Approximately 250 calories, 20g protein, 5g fat.

Lunch (3 PM):
Turkey and Vegetable Wrap with Whole Wheat Tortilla

- **Ingredients:**
  - 1 whole wheat tortilla
  - Turkey slices
  - Mixed vegetables (lettuce, tomatoes, cucumber)
  - Hummus for spreading

- **Instructions:**
  1. Lay out the tortilla.
  2. Spread hummus, add turkey slices, and top with mixed vegetables.
  3. Wrap and serve.

- **Nutrition:**
  - Approximately 350 calories, 18g protein, 12g fat.

Snack (6 PM):
Handful of Mixed Nuts

-Ingredients:
  - Almonds, walnuts, pistachios, etc.

- Instructions:
  - Enjoy a handful of mixed nuts.

- Nutrition:
  - Approximately 200 calories, 8g protein, 15g fat.

Dinner (8 PM):
Salmon and Asparagus Foil Pack

- Ingredients:
  - 1 salmon fillet
  - Asparagus spears
  - Lemon slices
  - Olive oil, garlic, and dill for seasoning

- Instructions:
  1. Place salmon, asparagus, and lemon slices on a foil sheet.

2. Drizzle with olive oil, season with garlic and dill, then fold into a foil pack.

3. Bake in the oven.

- Nutrition:

- Approximately 400 calories, 25g protein, 20g fat.
Certainly! Let's continue with the meal plan for the next few days:

DAY 3:

Breakfast (12 PM):
Chia Seed Pudding with Mixed Berries

- Ingredients:
- 2 tablespoons chia seeds
- 1 cup almond milk
- Mixed berries (strawberries, blueberries, raspberries)
- 1 tablespoon honey (optional)

-Instructions:
1. Mix chia seeds and almond milk, refrigerate overnight.

2. Top with mixed berries and drizzle with honey.

- Nutrition:
- Approximately 250 calories, 5g protein, 12g fat.

Lunch (3 PM):
Mediterranean Chickpea Salad

- Ingredients:
  - 1 can chickpeas, drained and rinsed
  - Cherry tomatoes, halved
  - Cucumber, diced
  - Red onion, finely chopped
  - Feta cheese, crumbled
  - Olive oil and balsamic vinegar dressing

- Instructions:
  1. Combine chickpeas, tomatoes, cucumber, red onion, and feta in a bowl.
  2. Drizzle with olive oil and balsamic vinegar.

- Nutrition:
  - Approximately 350 calories, 15g protein, 18g fat.

Snack (6 PM):
Hard-Boiled Eggs with a Dash of Salt

- Ingredients:
  - Hard-boiled eggs
  - Dash of salt

- Instructions:
  - Enjoy hard-boiled eggs with a dash of salt.

- **Nutrition:**
  - Approximately 150 calories, 12g protein, 10g fat.

Dinner (8 PM):
Vegetarian Stir-Fry with Tofu and Brown Rice

- **Ingredients:**
  - Tofu, cubed
  - Mixed vegetables (broccoli, bell peppers, snap peas)
  - Soy sauce, ginger, and garlic for seasoning
  - Cooked brown rice

-**Instructions:**
  1. Stir-fry tofu and vegetables with soy sauce, ginger, and garlic.
  2. Serve over cooked brown rice.

- **Nutrition:**
  - Approximately 400 calories, 20g protein, 15g fat.

DAY 4:

Breakfast (12 PM):
Whole Grain Toast with Smashed Avocado and Cherry Tomatoes

-**Ingredients:**

- 2 slices whole grain bread
- 1 avocado, smashed
- Cherry tomatoes, sliced
- Salt and pepper to taste

- Instructions:
1. Toast the bread.
2. Spread smashed avocado on the toast.
3. Top with sliced cherry tomatoes.
4. Season with salt and pepper.

- Nutrition:
- Approximately 300 calories, 8g protein, 15g fat.

Lunch (3 PM):
Quinoa and Black Bean Bowl with Salsa

- Ingredients:
- 1 cup cooked quinoa
- 1/2 cup black beans, drained and rinsed
- Corn kernels
- Salsa

- Instructions:
1. Combine quinoa, black beans, and corn in a bowl.
2. Top with salsa.

- Nutrition:

- Approximately 350 calories, 15g protein, 8g fat.

Snack (6 PM):
Orange Slices and a Handful of Almonds

- Ingredients:
  - Orange slices
  - Almonds

- Instructions:
  - Enjoy fresh orange slices with a handful of almonds.

- Nutrition:
  - Approximately 200 calories, 5g protein, 12g fat.

Dinner (8 PM):
Baked Cod with Roasted Vegetables and Quinoa

- Ingredients:
  - Cod filet
  - Assorted vegetables (zucchini, carrots, cherry tomatoes)
  - Olive oil, lemon, and herbs for seasoning
  - Cooked quinoa

- Instructions:
  1. Season cod with olive oil, lemon, and herbs, then bake.

2. Roast vegetables and serve over cooked quinoa.

- Nutrition:
  - Approximately 450 calories, 30g protein, 20g fat.

DAY 5:

Breakfast (12 PM):
Cottage Cheese with Pineapple and Sunflower Seeds

- Ingredients:
  - 1 cup low-fat cottage cheese
  - Fresh pineapple chunks
  - 1 tablespoon sunflower seeds

- Instructions:
  1. Combine cottage cheese with fresh pineapple.
  2. Sprinkle sunflower seeds on top.

- Nutrition:
  - Approximately 250 calories, 20g protein, 10g fat.

Lunch (3 PM):
Caprese Salad with Tomato, Mozzarella, and Basil

- Ingredients:
  - Tomatoes, sliced
  - Fresh mozzarella, sliced

- Fresh basil leaves
- Balsamic glaze

- Instructions:
1. Arrange tomato and mozzarella slices on a plate.
2. Garnish with fresh basil leaves and drizzle with balsamic glaze.

- Nutrition:
- Approximately 300 calories, 15g protein, 20g fat.

Snack (6 PM):
Handful of Mixed Nuts

- Ingredients:
- Almonds, walnuts, pistachios, etc.

- Instructions:
- Enjoy a handful of mixed nuts.

- Nutrition:
- Approximately 200 calories, 8g protein, 15g fat.

Dinner (8 PM):
Grilled Salmon with Asparagus and Quinoa

- Ingredients:
- Salmon fillet

- Fresh asparagus spears
- Lemon slices
- Olive oil, garlic, and herbs for seasoning
- Cooked quinoa

- Instructions:
1. Season salmon with olive oil, garlic, and herbs, then grill.
2. Grill asparagus alongside.
3. Serve over cooked quinoa.

- Nutrition:
- Approximately 400 calories, 30g protein, 20g fat.

DAY 6:

Breakfast (12 PM):
Chia Seed Pudding with Coconut Milk and Mixed Berries

- Ingredients:
- 2 tablespoons chia seeds
- 1 cup coconut milk
- Mixed berries (strawberries, blueberries, raspberries)

- Instructions:
1. Mix chia seeds and coconut milk, refrigerate overnight.

2. Top with mixed berries.

- Nutrition:
  - Approximately 250 calories, 5g protein, 15g fat.

Lunch (3 PM):
Turkey and Avocado Lettuce Wraps

- Ingredients:
  - Turkey slices
  - Avocado, sliced
  - Lettuce leaves

- Instructions:
  1. Lay out lettuce leaves.
  2. Add turkey slices and avocado, then wrap.

- Nutrition:
  - Approximately 300 calories, 20g protein, 15g fat.

Snack (6 PM):
Celery Sticks with Peanut Butter

- Ingredients:
  - Celery sticks
  - Peanut butter

- Instructions:

  - Spread peanut butter on celery sticks.

- Nutrition:
  - Approximately 150 calories, 5g protein, 10g fat.

Dinner (8 PM):
Baked Cod with Roasted Vegetables and Brown Rice

- Ingredients:
  - Cod fillet
  - Assorted vegetables (zucchini, carrots, cherry tomatoes)
  - Olive oil, lemon, and herbs for seasoning
  - Cooked brown rice

- Instructions:
  1. Season cod with olive oil, lemon, and herbs, then bake.
  2. Roast vegetables and serve over cooked brown rice.

- Nutrition:
  - Approximately 450 calories, 30g protein, 20g fat.

DAY 7:

Breakfast (12 PM):
Greek Yogurt Parfait with Granola and Mixed Berries

- **Ingredients:**
  - 1 cup Greek yogurt
  - Granola
  - Mixed berries (strawberries, blueberries, raspberries)

- **Instructions:**
  1. Layer Greek yogurt with granola and mixed berries in a bowl.

- **Nutrition:**
  - Approximately 300 calories, 15g protein, 10g fat.

Lunch (3 PM):
Vegetarian Buddha Bowl with Quinoa and Roasted Vegetables

- **Ingredients:**
  - 1 cup cooked quinoa
  - Roasted vegetables (sweet potatoes, Brussels sprouts, carrots)
  - Hummus
  - Avocado slices

- **Instructions:**
  1. Arrange quinoa, roasted vegetables, hummus, and avocado in a bowl.

- **Nutrition:**

- Approximately 350 calories, 12g protein, 15g fat.

Snack (6 PM):
Cucumber Slices with Tzatziki

- Ingredients:
  - Cucumber slices
  - Tzatziki sauce

- Instructions:
  - Dip cucumber slices in tzatziki sauce.

- Nutrition:
  - Approximately 100 calories, 5g protein, 5g fat.

Dinner (8 PM):
Grilled Shrimp with Lemon and Garlic, Served with Quinoa

- Ingredients:
  - Shrimp, peeled and deveined
  - Olive oil, lemon, and garlic for marinating
  - Cooked quinoa

- Instructions:
  1. Marinate shrimp in olive oil, lemon, and garlic, then grill.
  2. Serve over cooked quinoa.

- Nutrition:
  - Approximately 400 calories, 25g protein, 15g fat.

DAY 8:

Breakfast (12 PM):
Oatmeal with Almond Butter and Banana Slices

- Ingredients:
  - 1/2 cup oats
  - Almond butter
  - Banana slices

- Instructions:
  1. Cook oats according to package instructions.
  2. Top with almond butter and banana slices.

- Nutrition:
  - Approximately 300 calories, 10g protein, 12g fat.

Lunch (3 PM):
Chickpea and Spinach Salad with Feta Cheese

- Ingredients:
  - 1 can chickpeas, drained and rinsed
  - Fresh spinach leaves
  - Cherry tomatoes, halved

  - Feta cheese, crumbled
  - Olive oil and balsamic vinegar dressing

- Instructions:
1. Combine chickpeas, spinach, tomatoes, and feta in a bowl.
2. Drizzle with olive oil and balsamic vinegar.

- Nutrition:
  - Approximately 350 calories, 15g protein, 18g fat.

Snack (6 PM):
Yogurt-Covered Strawberries

- Ingredients:
  - Fresh strawberries
  - Greek yogurt

- Instructions:
1. Dip strawberries in Greek yogurt and freeze.

- Nutrition:
  - Approximately 150 calories, 5g protein, 8g fat.

Dinner (8 PM):
Baked Chicken Breast with Roasted Vegetables and Quinoa

- Ingredients:
  - Chicken breast
  - Assorted vegetables (bell peppers, broccoli, carrots)
  - Olive oil, garlic, and herbs for seasoning
  - Cooked quinoa

- Instructions:
  1. Season chicken with olive oil, garlic, and herbs, then bake.
  2. Roast vegetables and serve over cooked quinoa.

- Nutrition:
  - Approximately 450 calories, 30g protein, 20g fat.

DAY 9:

Breakfast (12 PM):
Egg White Omelette with Spinach, Tomato, and Feta

- Ingredients:
  - Egg whites
  - Fresh spinach
  - Tomato, diced
  - Feta cheese, crumbled

- Instructions:
  1. Cook egg whites and fold in spinach, tomatoes, and feta.

- **Nutrition:**
  - Approximately 250 calories, 20g protein, 10g fat.

Lunch (3 PM):
Quinoa and Vegetable Stuffed Bell Peppers

- **Ingredients:**
  - Bell peppers, halved
  - Quinoa and vegetable mix (broccoli, carrots, peas)
  - Tomato sauce

- **Instructions:**
  1. Fill bell peppers with quinoa and vegetable mix.
  2. Top with tomato sauce and bake.

- **Nutrition:**
  - Approximately 350 calories, 15g protein, 18g fat.

Snack (6 PM):
Trail Mix with Nuts and Dried Fruits

- **Ingredients:**
  - Almonds, walnuts, dried cranberries, raisins, etc.

- **Instructions:**
  - Combine nuts and dried fruits for a trail mix.

- Nutrition:
  - Approximately 200 calories, 8g protein, 12g fat.

Dinner (8 PM):
Baked Cod with Lemon and Herb Quinoa

- Ingredients:
  - Cod fillet
  - Lemon and herb marinade
  - Cooked quinoa

- Instructions:
  1. Marinate cod in lemon and herb mixture, then bake.
  2. Serve over cooked quinoa.

- Nutrition:
  - Approximately 400 calories, 25g protein, 15g fat.

DAY 10:

Breakfast (12 PM):
Smoothie Bowl with Mixed Berries, Almond Milk, and Granola

- Ingredients:
  - Mixed berries
  - Almond milk
  - Granola

- Instructions:
  1. Blend mixed berries with almond milk.
  2. Top with granola.

- Nutrition:
  - Approximately 300 calories, 10g protein, 15g fat.

Lunch (3 PM):
Turkey and Quinoa Stuffed Zucchini Boats

- Ingredients:
  - Zucchini, halved
  - Ground turkey
  - Quinoa
  - Tomato sauce

- Instructions:
  1. Hollow out zucchini and stuff with a mixture of ground turkey and quinoa.
  2. Top with tomato sauce and bake.

- Nutrition:
  - Approximately 350 calories, 20g protein, 15g fat.

Snack (6 PM):
Greek Yogurt with Sliced Kiwi

- **Ingredients:**
  - Greek yogurt
  - Kiwi, sliced

- **Instructions**:
  - Enjoy Greek yogurt with sliced kiwi.

- **Nutrition:**
  - Approximately 150 calories, 12g protein, 8g fat.

Dinner (8 PM):
Grilled Chicken Salad with Avocado and Balsamic
Vinaigrette

- **Ingredients:**
  - Grilled chicken breast
  - Mixed greens
  - Avocado, sliced
  - Balsamic vinaigrette dressing

- **Instructions:**
  1. Toss grilled chicken, mixed greens, and avocado.
  2. Drizzle with balsamic vinaigrette.

- **Nutrition:**
  - Approximately 450 calories, 30g protein, 20g fat.

DAY 11:

Breakfast (12 PM):
Peanut Butter and Banana Smoothie

- Ingredients:
  - 1 banana
  - 2 tablespoons peanut butter
  - 1 cup almond milk
  - Ice cubes

- Instructions:
  1. Blend banana, peanut butter, almond milk, and ice cubes until smooth.

- Nutrition:
  - Approximately 300 calories, 10g protein, 15g fat.

Lunch (3 PM):
Mediterranean Quinoa Bowl with Hummus

- Ingredients:
  - 1 cup cooked quinoa
  - Cherry tomatoes, halved
  - Cucumber, diced
  - Kalamata olives
  - Feta cheese
  - Hummus

- Instructions:

  1. Mix quinoa, tomatoes, cucumber, olives, and feta in a bowl.

  2. Top with a dollop of hummus.

- Nutrition:

  - Approximately 350 calories, 15g protein, 18g fat.

Snack (6 PM):

Homemade Energy Bites

- Ingredients:

  - Oats, almond butter, honey, chia seeds, dark chocolate chips

- Instructions:

  1. Combine ingredients and form into small energy bites.

- Nutrition:

  - Approximately 200 calories, 8g protein, 12g fat.

Dinner (8 PM):

Vegetarian Stir-Fry with Tofu and Brown Rice

- Ingredients:

  - Tofu, cubed
  - Mixed vegetables (broccoli, bell peppers, snap peas)

- Soy sauce, ginger, and garlic for seasoning
- Cooked brown rice

- Instructions:
1. Stir-fry tofu and vegetables with soy sauce, ginger, and garlic.
2. Serve over cooked brown rice.

- Nutrition:
- Approximately 400 calories, 20g protein, 15g fat.

DAY 12:

Breakfast (12 PM):
Yogurt Parfait with Granola and Mixed Berries

- Ingredients:
- Greek yogurt
- Granola
- Mixed berries (strawberries, blueberries, raspberries)

- Instructions:
1. Layer Greek yogurt with granola and mixed berries in a glass.

- Nutrition:
- Approximately 300 calories, 15g protein, 10g fat.

Lunch (3 PM):
Salmon and Avocado Wrap

- Ingredients:
  - Grilled salmon
  - Whole wheat wrap
  - Avocado slices
  - Lettuce, tomato

- Instructions:
  1. Fill the whole wheat wrap with grilled salmon, avocado, lettuce, and tomato.

- Nutrition:
  - Approximately 350 calories, 20g protein, 15g fat.

Snack (6 PM):
Cottage Cheese with Pineapple

- Ingredients:
  - Cottage cheese
  - Fresh pineapple chunks

- Instructions:
  - Combine cottage cheese with fresh pineapple.

- Nutrition:
  - Approximately 200 calories, 15g protein, 10g fat.

Dinner (8 PM):
Chicken and Vegetable Skewers with Quinoa

- Ingredients:
  - Chicken breast, cubed
  - Assorted vegetables (bell peppers, onions, cherry tomatoes)
  - Olive oil, lemon, and herbs for seasoning
  - Cooked quinoa

- Instructions:
  1. Thread chicken and vegetables onto skewers.
  2. Grill or bake, then serve over cooked quinoa.

- Nutrition:
  - Approximately 450 calories, 30g protein, 20g fat.

DAY 13:

Breakfast (12 PM):
Vegetarian Breakfast Burrito

- Ingredients:
  - Scrambled eggs or tofu
  - Black beans
  - Avocado slices
  - Whole wheat tortilla

- Instructions:

1. Fill a whole wheat tortilla with scrambled eggs or tofu, black beans, and avocado slices.

- Nutrition:

- Approximately 300 calories, 15g protein, 15g fat.

Lunch (3 PM):
Quinoa Salad with Chickpeas and Feta

- Ingredients:
- 1 cup cooked quinoa
- Chickpeas, drained and rinsed
- Cherry tomatoes, halved
- Feta cheese, crumbled
- Lemon vinaigrette dressing

- Instructions:

1. Combine quinoa, chickpeas, tomatoes, and feta in a bowl.
2. Drizzle with lemon vinaigrette dressing.

- Nutrition:

- Approximately 350 calories, 15g protein, 18g fat.

Snack (6 PM):
Mixed Berries with Greek Yogurt

- Ingredients:
  - Mixed berries
  - Greek yogurt

- Instructions:
  - Enjoy a bowl of mixed berries with a dollop of Greek yogurt.

- Nutrition:
  - Approximately 150 calories, 8g protein, 5g fat.

Dinner (8 PM):
Baked Halibut with Roasted Vegetables and Quinoa

- Ingredients:
  - Halibut fillet
  - Assorted vegetables (zucchini, carrots, bell peppers)
  - Olive oil, lemon, and herbs for seasoning
  - Cooked quinoa

- Instructions:
  1. Season halibut with olive oil, lemon, and herbs, then bake.
  2. Roast vegetables and serve over cooked quinoa.

- Nutrition:
  - Approximately 400 calories, 25g protein, 15g fat.

DAY 14:

Breakfast (12 PM):
Blueberry Protein Pancakes

- Ingredients:
  - Whole grain pancake mix
  - Blueberries
  - Greek yogurt topping

- Instructions:
  1. Prepare pancakes with whole grain mix, adding blueberries.
  2. Top with a dollop of Greek yogurt.

- Nutrition:
  - Approximately 300 calories, 15g protein, 10g fat.

Lunch (3 PM):
Spinach and Mushroom Frittata

- Ingredients:
  - Eggs
  - Spinach
  - Mushrooms
  - Feta cheese

- Instructions:

1. Cook eggs with spinach, mushrooms, and feta to make a frittata.

- Nutrition:

- Approximately 350 calories, 20g protein, 18g fat.

Snack (6 PM):

Handful of Almonds and Dried Apricots

- Ingredients:

- Almonds
- Dried apricots

- Instructions:

- Combine almonds with dried apricots for a satisfying snack.

- Nutrition:

- Approximately 200 calories, 8g protein, 12g fat.

Dinner (8 PM):

Turkey and Vegetable Stir-Fry with Brown Rice

- Ingredients:

- Ground turkey
- Mixed vegetables (broccoli, bell peppers, snap peas)
- Soy sauce, ginger, and garlic for seasoning

- Cooked brown rice

- Instructions:
   1. Stir-fry ground turkey and vegetables with soy sauce, ginger, and garlic.
   2. Serve over cooked brown rice.

- Nutrition:
   - Approximately 450 calories, 30g protein, 20g fat.

DAY 15:

Breakfast (12 PM):
Avocado and Egg Toast

- Ingredients:
   - Whole grain toast
   - Avocado slices
   - Poached or fried egg
   - Salt and pepper to taste

-Instructions:
   1. Spread avocado on whole grain toast and top with a poached or fried egg.
   2. Season with salt and pepper.

- Nutrition:
   - Approximately 300 calories, 15g protein, 15g fat.

Lunch (3 PM):
Chickpea and Vegetable Wrap

- Ingredients:
  - Whole wheat wrap
  - Chickpeas, mashed
  - Mixed vegetables (cucumber, bell peppers, tomatoes)
  - Hummus

- Instructions:
  1. Spread mashed chickpeas on a whole wheat wrap.
  2. Add mixed vegetables and a dollop of hummus, then
wrap.

- Nutrition:
  - Approximately 350 calories, 15g protein, 18g fat.

Snack (6 PM):
Cucumber and Hummus Slices

- Ingredients:
  - Cucumber slices
  - Hummus

- Instructions:
  - Dip cucumber slices in hummus.

- Nutrition:
  - Approximately 100 calories, 5g protein, 5g fat.

Dinner (8 PM):
Salmon and Quinoa Bowl with Roasted Vegetables

- Ingredients:
  - Grilled salmon
  - 1 cup cooked quinoa
  - Roasted vegetables (zucchini, cherry tomatoes, asparagus)
  - Lemon-tahini dressing

- Instructions:
  1. Assemble grilled salmon, cooked quinoa, and roasted vegetables in a bowl.
  2. Drizzle with lemon-tahini dressing.

- Nutrition:
  - Approximately 400 calories, 25g protein, 15g fat.

DAY 16:

Breakfast (12 PM):
Smoothie with Kale, Banana, and Protein Powder

- Ingredients:
  - Kale leaves

- Banana
- Protein powder
- Almond milk

- Instructions:

1. Blend kale, banana, protein powder, and almond milk until smooth.

- Nutrition:

- Approximately 300 calories, 20g protein, 10g fat.

Lunch (3 PM):

Shrimp and Avocado Salad

- Ingredients:

- Grilled shrimp
- Mixed greens
- Avocado slices
- Cherry tomatoes
- Balsamic vinaigrette dressing

- Instructions:

1. Toss grilled shrimp, mixed greens, avocado slices, and cherry tomatoes.
2. Drizzle with balsamic vinaigrette.

- Nutrition:

- Approximately 350 calories, 20g protein, 15g fat.

Snack (6 PM):
Greek Yogurt with Mango Slices

- Ingredients:
  - Greek yogurt
  - Fresh mango slices

- Instructions:
  - Enjoy Greek yogurt with fresh mango slices.

- Nutrition:
  - Approximately 150 calories, 12g protein, 8g fat.

Dinner (8 PM):
Vegetarian Lentil and Vegetable Stew

- Ingredients:
  - Lentils
  - Mixed vegetables (carrots, celery, onions)
  - Vegetable broth
  - Herbs and spices for seasoning

- Instructions:
  1. Cook lentils and mixed vegetables in vegetable broth.
  2. Season with herbs and spices.

- **Nutrition:**
  - Approximately 400 calories, 20g protein, 15g fat.

DAY 17:

Breakfast (12 PM):
Chia Seed Pudding with Berries

- **Ingredients:**
  - Chia seeds
  - Almond milk
  - Mixed berries

- **Instructions:**
  1. Mix chia seeds with almond milk and let it sit overnight to form a pudding.
  2. Top with mixed berries.

- **Nutrition:**
  - Approximately 300 calories, 10g protein, 15g fat.

Lunch (3 PM):
Grilled Chicken Caesar Salad

- **Ingredients:**
  - Grilled chicken breast
  - Romaine lettuce
  - Cherry tomatoes

- Parmesan cheese
- Caesar dressing

- Instructions:
1. Toss grilled chicken, romaine lettuce, cherry tomatoes, and Parmesan cheese.
2. Drizzle with Caesar dressing.

- Nutrition:
- Approximately 350 calories, 25g protein, 15g fat.

Snack (6 PM):
Whole Grain Crackers with Guacamole

- Ingredients:
- Whole grain crackers
- Guacamole

- Instructions:
- Enjoy whole grain crackers with guacamole.

- Nutrition:
- Approximately 150 calories, 5g protein, 10g fat.

Dinner (8 PM):
Vegetarian Stuffed Bell Peppers

- Ingredients:

- Bell peppers, halved
- Quinoa and black bean mix
- Salsa
- Shredded cheese

- Instructions:
1. Fill bell peppers with quinoa and black bean mix.
2. Top with salsa and shredded cheese, then bake.

- Nutrition:
- Approximately 400 calories, 15g protein, 20g fat.

DAY 18:

Breakfast (12 PM):
Omelette with Spinach, Tomato, and Feta

- Ingredients:
- Eggs
- Fresh spinach
- Tomato, diced
- Feta cheese, crumbled

- Instructions:
1. Cook eggs and fold in spinach, tomatoes, and feta.

- Nutrition:
- Approximately 300 calories, 15g protein, 15g fat.

Lunch (3 PM):
Turkey and Quinoa Salad Bowl

- Ingredients:
  - Turkey slices
  - 1 cup cooked quinoa
  - Mixed greens
  - Cucumber, diced
  - Lemon-tahini dressing

- Instructions:
  1. Arrange turkey slices, cooked quinoa, mixed greens, and diced cucumber in a bowl.
  2. Drizzle with lemon-tahini dressing.

- Nutrition:
  - Approximately 350 calories, 20g protein, 15g fat.

Snack (6 PM):
Cottage Cheese with Pineapple

- Ingredients:
  - Cottage cheese
  - Fresh pineapple chunks

- Instructions:
  - Combine cottage cheese with fresh pineapple.

- Nutrition:
  - Approximately 200 calories, 15g protein, 10g fat.

Dinner (8 PM):
Baked Cod with Lemon and Herb Couscous

- Ingredients:
  - Cod fillet
  - Lemon and herb marinade
  - Cooked couscous

- Instructions:
  1. Marinate cod in lemon and herb mixture, then bake.
  2. Serve over cooked couscous.

- Nutrition:
  - Approximately 400 calories, 25g protein, 15g fat.

DAY 19:

Breakfast (12 PM):
Greek Yogurt Parfait with Granola and Berries

- Ingredients:
  - Greek yogurt
  - Granola
  - Mixed berries (strawberries, blueberries, raspberries)

- **Instructions:**

1. Layer Greek yogurt with granola and mixed berries in a glass.

- **Nutrition:**

- Approximately 300 calories, 15g protein, 10g fat.

Lunch (3 PM):
Caprese Salad with Balsamic Glaze

- **Ingredients:**
  - Fresh mozzarella
  - Tomatoes, sliced
  - Fresh basil leaves
  - Balsamic glaze

- **Instructions:**

1. Arrange fresh mozzarella, sliced tomatoes, and basil leaves on a plate.
2. Drizzle with balsamic glaze.

- **Nutrition:**

- Approximately 350 calories, 20g protein, 20g fat.

Snack (6 PM):
Mixed Nuts and Dried Fruit

- Ingredients:
  - Almonds, walnuts, dried cranberries, raisins, etc.

- Instructions:
  - Combine a variety of nuts and dried fruits for a nutritious snack.

- Nutrition:
  - Approximately 200 calories, 8g protein, 12g fat.

Dinner (8 PM):
Stuffed Portobello Mushrooms with Quinoa and Vegetables

- Ingredients:
  - Portobello mushrooms
  - Quinoa and vegetable stuffing
  - Olive oil, herbs, and spices

- Instructions:
  1. Fill portobello mushrooms with quinoa and vegetable stuffing.
  2. Drizzle with olive oil and season with herbs and spices, then bake.

- Nutrition:
  - Approximately 400 calories, 20g protein, 15g fat.

DAY 20:

Breakfast (12 PM):
Pumpkin Spice Overnight Oats

- **Ingredients:**
  - Rolled oats
  - Almond milk
  - Pumpkin puree
  - Maple syrup and cinnamon for flavor

- **Instructions:**
  1. Mix rolled oats, almond milk, pumpkin puree, maple syrup, and cinnamon.
  2. Let it sit overnight in the refrigerator.

- **Nutrition:**
  - Approximately 300 calories, 10g protein, 15g fat.

Lunch (3 PM):
Chicken and Vegetable Wrap

- **Ingredients:**
  - Grilled chicken strips
  - Whole wheat wrap
  - Mixed vegetables (bell peppers, onions)
  - Greek yogurt sauce

- Instructions:

1. Fill a whole wheat wrap with grilled chicken, mixed vegetables, and a Greek yogurt sauce.

- Nutrition:

  - Approximately 350 calories, 25g protein, 15g fat.

Snack (6 PM):
Apple Slices with Almond Butter

- Ingredients:

  - Apple, sliced
  - Almond butter

- Instructions:

  - Dip apple slices in almond butter.

- Nutrition:

  - Approximately 150 calories, 5g protein, 10g fat.

Dinner (8 PM):
Vegetarian Lentil and Sweet Potato Curry

- Ingredients:

  - Lentils
  - Sweet potatoes, diced
  - Coconut milk
  - Curry spices

- Instructions:

1. Cook lentils and sweet potatoes in coconut milk with curry spices.

2. Serve over rice or quinoa.

- Nutrition:

- Approximately 400 calories, 20g protein, 15g fat.

DAY 21:

Breakfast (12 PM):

Avocado and Tomato Toast with Poached Egg

- Ingredients:
  - 1 slice whole-grain bread
  - 1/2 avocado, mashed
  - 1 tomato, sliced
  - 1 poached egg
  - Salt and pepper to taste

- Instructions:
  1. Toast the bread.
  2. Spread mashed avocado on the toast.
  3. Top with tomato slices and a poached egg.
  4. Season with salt and pepper.

- Nutrition:

- Approximately 300 calories, 15g protein, 15g fat.

Lunch (3 PM):
Quinoa Salad with Chickpeas, Cucumber, and Feta

- Ingredients:
  - 1 cup cooked quinoa
  - 1/2 cup chickpeas, drained and rinsed
  - 1 cucumber, diced
  - 1/4 cup feta cheese, crumbled
  - Olive oil and lemon dressing

- **Instructions:**
  1. In a bowl, combine quinoa, chickpeas, cucumber, and feta.
  2. Drizzle with olive oil and lemon dressing.

- **Nutrition:**
  - Approximately 350 calories, 12g protein, 15g fat.

Snack (6 PM):
Greek Yogurt with Berries and a Drizzle of Honey

- **Ingredients**:
  - 1 cup Greek yogurt
  - Mixed berries (strawberries, blueberries, raspberries)
  - 1 tablespoon honey

- **Instructions**:
  1. In a bowl, mix Greek yogurt with berries.
  2. Drizzle with honey.

- **Nutrition:**
  - Approximately 200 calories, 15g protein, 5g fat.

Dinner (8 PM):
Grilled Chicken Breast with Roasted Vegetables and Sweet Potato

- **ingredients**:
  - 1 boneless, skinless chicken breast
  - Assorted vegetables (bell peppers, zucchini, cherry tomatoes)
  - 1 sweet potato, diced
  - Olive oil, garlic, and herbs for seasoning

- **Instructions:**
  1. Season the chicken breast with olive oil, garlic, and herbs, then grill.
  2. Roast vegetables and sweet potatoes in the oven.

- **Nutrition:**
  - Approximately 400 calories, 30g protein, 15g fat.

DAY 22:

Breakfast (12 PM):
Smoothie with Spinach, Banana, and Protein Powder

-Ingredients:
  - 1 cup spinach
  - 1 banana
  - 1 scoop protein powder
  - 1 cup almond milk

- Instructions:
  1. Blend all ingredients until smooth.

- **Nutrition**:
  - Approximately 250 calories, 20g protein, 5g fat.

Lunch (3 PM):
Turkey and Vegetable Wrap with Whole Wheat Tortilla

- **Ingredients**:
  - 1 whole wheat tortilla
  - Turkey slices
  - Mixed vegetables (lettuce, tomatoes, cucumber)
  - Hummus for spreading

- **Instructions:**
  1. Lay out the tortilla.
  2. Spread hummus, add turkey slices, and top with mixed vegetables.

3. Wrap and serve.

- **Nutrition**:
  - Approximately 350 calories, 18g protein, 12g fat.

Snack (6 PM):
Handful of Mixed Nuts

- **Ingredients**:
  - Almonds, walnuts, pistachios, etc.

- **Instructions**:
  - Enjoy a handful of mixed nuts.

- **Nutrition**:
  - Approximately 200 calories, 8g protein, 15g fat.

Dinner (8 PM):
Salmon and Asparagus Foil Pack

- **Ingredients:**
  - 1 salmon filet
  - Asparagus spears
  - Lemon slices
  - Olive oil, garlic, and dill for seasoning

- **Instructions**:

  1. Place salmon, asparagus, and lemon slices on a foil
sheet.
  2. Drizzle with olive oil, season with garlic and dill,
then fold into a foil pack.
  3. Bake in the oven.

- **Nutrition:**
  - Approximately 400 calories, 25g protein, 20g fat.

DAY 23:

Breakfast (12 PM):
Greek Yogurt Parfait with Mixed Berries and Almonds

- **Ingredients**:
  - 1 cup Greek yogurt
  - Mixed berries (strawberries, blueberries, raspberries)
  - 1/4 cup almonds, sliced

- **Instructions**:
  1. Layer Greek yogurt with mixed berries in a bowl.
  2. Top with sliced almonds.

- **Nutrition**:
  - Approximately 350 calories, 20g protein, 15g fat.

Lunch (3 PM):

Grilled Chicken Salad with Avocado and Olive Oil Dressing

- **Ingredients**:
  - Grilled chicken breast
  - Mixed salad greens
  - Cherry tomatoes
  - Avocado, sliced
  - Olive oil dressing

- **Instructions**:
  1. Combine grilled chicken, salad greens, cherry tomatoes, and avocado in a bowl.
  2. Drizzle with olive oil dressing.

- **Nutrition**:
  - Approximately 400 calories, 25g protein, 20g fat.

Snack (6 PM):
Apple Slices with Almond Butter

- **Ingredients:**
  - 1 apple, sliced
  - Almond butter

- **Instructions**:
  1. Dip apple slices in almond butter.

- **Nutrition**:
  - Approximately 150 calories, 3g protein, 8g fat.

Dinner (8 PM):
Baked Salmon with Roasted Brussels Sprouts and
Quinoa

- **Ingredients:**
  - Salmon filet
  - Brussels sprouts
  - Quinoa
  - Olive oil, lemon, and herbs for seasoning

- **Instructions:**
  1. Season salmon with olive oil, lemon, and herbs, then
bake.
  2. Roast Brussels sprouts.
  3. Serve over cooked quinoa.

- **Nutrition:**
  - Approximately 450 calories, 30g protein, 20g fat.

DAY 24:

Breakfast (12 PM):
Avocado and Tomato Toast

- **Ingredients:**

- 1 slice whole-grain bread
- 1/2 ripe avocado
- Sliced tomatoes
- Salt and pepper to taste

- **Instructions:**
  1. Toast the whole-grain bread.
  2. Mash the avocado and spread it on the toast.
  3. Top with sliced tomatoes and season with salt and pepper.

- **Nutrition:**
  - Approximately 250 calories, 5g protein, 15g fat.

Lunch (3 PM):
Grilled Chicken Salad

- Ingredients:
  - Grilled chicken breast
  - Mixed salad greens
  - Cherry tomatoes
  - Cucumber slices
  - Olive oil and balsamic vinaigrette

- **Instructions**:
  1. Combine grilled chicken, salad greens, cherry tomatoes, and cucumber slices.

2. Drizzle with a mixture of olive oil and balsamic vinaigrette.

- **Nutrition:**
  - Approximately 300 calories, 25g protein, 12g fat.

Dinner (8 PM):
Salmon with Roasted Vegetables

- **Ingredients:**
  - Salmon filet
  - Assorted vegetables (broccoli, carrots, bell peppers)
  - Olive oil, garlic, and herbs

- **Instructions:**
  1. Season the salmon with herbs and bake.
  2. Roast assorted vegetables with olive oil and garlic.

- **Nutrition:**
  - Approximately 400 calories, 30g protein, 20g fat.

DAY 25:

Breakfast (12 PM):
Greek Yogurt Parfait

- **Ingredients:**
  - Greek yogurt

- Mixed berries (strawberries, blueberries)
- Granola

- Instructions:
1. Layer Greek yogurt with mixed berries and granola.

- Nutrition:
- Approximately 280 calories, 15g protein, 10g fat.

Lunch (3 PM):
Quinoa and Chickpea Salad

- Ingredients:
- Cooked quinoa
- Chickpeas
- Cherry tomatoes
- Cucumber, diced
- Feta cheese
- Lemon vinaigrette

- Instructions:
1. Combine quinoa, chickpeas, cherry tomatoes, cucumber, and feta cheese.
2. Drizzle with lemon vinaigrette.

- Nutrition:
- Approximately 350 calories, 18g protein, 15g fat.

Dinner (8 PM):
Vegetarian Stir-Fry with Tofu

- **Ingredients:**
  - Tofu, cubed
  - Mixed stir-fry vegetables (broccoli, bell peppers, snap peas)
  - Soy sauce, ginger, and garlic

- **Instructions**:
  1. Stir-fry tofu and vegetables with soy sauce, ginger, and garlic.

- **Nutrition**:
  - Approximately 380 calories, 20g protein, 18g fat.

DAY 26:

Breakfast (12 PM):
Berry Protein Smoothie

- **Ingredients:**
  - Mixed berries (strawberries, raspberries, blueberries)
  - Protein powder
  - Almond milk

- **Instructions**:

1. Blend mixed berries, protein powder, and almond milk.

- **Nutrition**:
  - Approximately 250 calories, 20g protein, 10g fat.

Lunch (3 PM):
Turkey and Avocado Wrap

- **Ingredients**:
  - Whole-grain wrap
  - Sliced turkey breast
  - Avocado slices
  - Lettuce and tomato

- **Instructions:**
  1. Fill a whole-grain wrap with turkey, avocado, lettuce, and tomato.

- **Nutrition:**
  - Approximately 320 calories, 25g protein, 15g fat.

Dinner (8 PM):
Baked Cod with Lemon and Herbs

- **Ingredients:**
  - Cod filet
  - Lemon juice, olive oil, and herbs

- Instructions:
   1. Marinate cod with lemon juice, olive oil, and herbs.
   2. Bake until cooked through.

- Nutrition:
   - Approximately 350 calories, 30g protein, 18g fat.

DAY 27:

Breakfast (12 PM):
Egg and Vegetable Omelet

- Ingredients:
   - Eggs
   - Bell peppers, onions, spinach
   - Feta cheese

- Instructions:
   1. Whisk eggs and pour over sautéed vegetables.
   2. Sprinkle with feta cheese and cook until set.

- Nutrition:
   - Approximately 280 calories, 18g protein, 15g fat.

Lunch (3 PM):
Spinach and Chickpea Soup

- **Ingredients**:
  - Spinach
  - Chickpeas
  - Vegetable broth
  - Garlic, onion, and spices

- **Instructions:**
  1. Sauté garlic and onion, add spinach, chickpeas, and vegetable broth.
  2. Simmer until flavors meld.

- **Nutrition:**
  - Approximately 300 calories, 15g protein, 10g fat.

Dinner (8 PM):
Grilled Shrimp Skewers with Quinoa

- **Ingredients:**
  - Shrimp
  - Quinoa
  - Lemon, olive oil, and herbs

- **Instructions**:
  1. Marinate shrimp in lemon, olive oil, and herbs.
  2. Grill shrimp and serve over cooked quinoa.

- **Nutrition:**
  - Approximately 400 calories, 25g protein, 20g fat.

DAY 28:

Breakfast (12 PM):
Peanut Butter Banana Smoothie

- **Ingredients:**
  - Banana
  - Peanut butter
  - Greek yogurt
  - Almond milk

- **Instructions:**
  1. Blend banana, peanut butter, Greek yogurt, and almond milk.

- **Nutrition:**
  - Approximately 300 calories, 15g protein, 15g fat.

Lunch (3 PM):
Mediterranean Salad with Chicken

- **Ingredients:**
  - Grilled chicken strips
  - Mixed greens
  - Cherry tomatoes, olives, feta cheese
  - Olive oil and balsamic vinaigrette

- **Instructions:**

   1. Combine grilled chicken, mixed greens, tomatoes, olives, and feta cheese.

   2. Drizzle with olive oil and balsamic vinaigrette.

- **Nutrition:**

   - Approximately 350 calories, 30g protein, 15g fat.

Dinner (8 PM):

Vegetable and Lentil Stew

- **Ingredients:**

   - Lentils
   - Assorted vegetables (carrots, celery, tomatoes)
   - Vegetable broth, garlic, and herbs

- **Instructions:**

   1. Cook lentils with vegetables, garlic, and herbs in vegetable broth.

- **Nutrition:**

   - Approximately 380 calories, 20g protein, 18g fat.

CONCLUSION

Finally, the value of intermittent fasting for women over 50 cannot be emphasized, as it seems to be a potential route for boosting general health and well-being at this critical life stage. As we consider the numerous factors discussed, it becomes clear that intermittent fasting provides a diverse strategy to tackling the particular health concerns that women in this group confront.

1. Metabolic Health and Weight Management:
Intermittent fasting shows potential benefits in enhancing metabolic health and managing weight, crucial considerations for women over 50 who may experience shifts in metabolism and body composition. By regulating calorie intake and promoting fat loss while preserving lean muscle mass, intermittent fasting can contribute to a healthier and more resilient body.

2. Hormonal Considerations:
Understanding the hormonal landscape during menopause is essential, and intermittent fasting can be tailored to address these considerations. The potential positive impact on insulin sensitivity and hormonal balance may offer women over 50 a valuable tool in navigating the changes associated with this life stage.

3. Cognitive Well-Being:

The potential neuroprotective effects of intermittent fasting, particularly in promoting the production of brain-derived neurotrophic factor (BDNF), underscore its significance in supporting cognitive well-being. As cognitive health becomes a prominent concern with age, strategies that may contribute to maintaining brain function are of utmost importance.

4. Long-Term Health and Chronic Disease Prevention:
The long-term health implications of intermittent fasting extend beyond the immediate benefits. Evidence suggests that adopting intermittent fasting may contribute to a decreased risk of chronic diseases such as diabetes and cardiovascular issues. This preventive aspect is particularly relevant for women over 50 aiming to safeguard their health in the years to come.

5. Individualization and Sustainable Lifestyle:
Recognizing the individualized nature of health journeys, intermittent fasting allows for flexibility and adaptability. It can be tailored to suit different lifestyles, preferences, and health goals, emphasizing the importance of adopting practices that are sustainable for the long term. This individualized approach is essential for ensuring the adherence and success of intermittent fasting regimens.

6. Positive Impact on Nutritional Choices:

Intermittent fasting encourages a mindful approach to eating, fostering an awareness of nutritional choices during eating windows. By emphasizing nutrient-dense foods and discouraging unhealthy eating habits, intermittent fasting promotes a positive impact on overall dietary patterns, contributing to better nutritional outcomes for women over 50.

7. Empowerment and Well-Being:
Engaging in intermittent fasting can empower women over 50 to take an active role in their health and well-being. By understanding the principles of intermittent fasting and its potential benefits, women can make informed decisions about their lifestyle and dietary choices, fostering a sense of empowerment and control over their health.

Basically, intermittent fasting for women over 50 is consistent with a proactive and comprehensive approach to health. It extends beyond food limitations to include a range of physical, hormonal, and mental well-being. While acknowledging the potential components of intermittent fasting, women must approach this lifestyle choice with caution, talking with healthcare specialists, and putting it within a larger framework of good living.

As research in this field continues to unfold, women over 50 are encouraged to stay informed, remain attuned to their bodies, and make choices that resonate with their unique health journeys. Intermittent fasting stands as a tool that, when utilized mindfully and tailored to individual needs, can contribute significantly to the overall health and vitality of women as they navigate the enriching years beyond 50.